"Currently about fifty percent of all pregnancies are either unwanted or unplanned, and that is why the hope and inspiration provided by Jill Hopkins in *Welcoming the Soul of a Child* is so urgently needed. This precious book lights the way for all those who have the courage and clarity to consciously welcome their children into this world even before they are conceived—and by doing so, heal themselves."
—Christiane Northrup, M.D., author of
Women's Bodies, Women's Wisdom

"A wonderful and insightful book, *Welcoming the Soul of a Child* gives couples a starting place in their journey of preparation toward parenthood, a journey that will be the most important one of their lives. It is vitally important that we view each and every being in a sacred and loving way, and Jill Hopkins has just given us a road map from which to begin."
—Barbara Harper, R.N., author of *Gentle Birth Choices*

"Tender, wise, and practical, *Welcoming the Soul of a Child* is a book that every parent-to-be will cherish. Bringing the sacred back to conception and birth is a critical step for curbing the escalating violence in our culture and cultivating the compassion that is our true nature."
—Joan Borysenko, Ph.D., author of *A Woman's Book of Life*

"Birth is a critical point in the life of the soul as well as the body. This quietly engaging and practical book guides us from soul-wounding to soul-welcoming behavior . . . and invites us to a deeper appreciation of the great and unique value of each human being."
—Thomas R. Yeomans, author of *The Soul Wound*

"Going beyond obstetrics, beyond psychology, and beyond childbirth education, Jill Hopkins give us the first handbook for couples seeking the ultimate spiritual challenge: parenting a soul. Her brand of spirituality is sensitively ecumenical, cross-cultural, and user-friendly."

'h.D., author of
Newborn Baby

WELCOMING THE SOUL OF A CHILD

Jill E. Hopkins

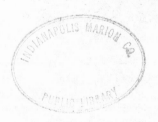

Kensington Books
http://www.kensingtonbooks.com

For Zach,
and the song of his soul

KENSINGTON BOOKS are published by

Kensington Publishing Corp.
850 Third Avenue
New York, NY 10022

Kensington and the K logo Reg. U.S. Pat. & TM Off.

ISBN 1-57566-428-3

First Printing: May, 1999
10 9 8 7 6 5 4 3 2 1

Printed in the United States of America

Verny—it is truly an honor to have your good wishes and support for this book's message. Thank you.

Heartfelt thanks to my entire family. Warm love to Bette for *always* being there when we need you. Fondest love to my mother Dorothy and father Bill.

Special acknowledgment to my friends, who not only reminded me, but encouraged me to breathe, move my body, howl, cry and laugh during the process of birthing this book. Loving gratitude always to Linda Logan, Dea Shandera, Leesa Sklover-Filgate, Charla Brown, Rob Burnett, Jeanne Barrett and Marty Spiegel. Affectionate love, especially to Marcia Bernstein, Ken and Marilynn Balter and Jeff and Diane Rossman, who after reading my earliest scribbles urged me to keep writing.

Deepest appreciation to each and every individual who shared her or his intimate story. For it is these stories that provide the silk and satin threads that lovingly hold and carry the heart of this writing to you, the reader.

To Steven, for wrapping your wonderful arms around me (and the book) throughout all of the stages of this labor of love. I will always love you.

And to Zachary, whose soul's song inspires me every day. I am truly blessed to have you in my life. May you come to know this book as a humble gift of love for you and all children everywhere.

Acknowledgments

From the very beginning it has felt like this book has had a soul with a song to sing. I feel blessed for the community of extraordinary people who have welcomed and honored that song into being.

Profound gratitude to Jack Kornfield for his inspiring generosity of heart and for blessing this book from its earliest days.

To Stephen and Ondrea Levine, who must have heard the book's soul singing all the way up in the mountains of New Mexico. Deepest appreciation for your wisdom and lovely words.

Warmest thanks to Thomas Yeomans for his encouragement and rich teachings, especially those around the soul wound.

I am grateful to Jane Dystel for being there soon after the idea of the book was conceived and for nurturing that idea along.

Deepest thanks to Tracy Bernstein at Kensington Publishing for enthusiastically and tenderly welcoming the heart and soul of this material.

Stephanie Jourdan, spiritual midwife, guide and friend— thank you always for helping me believe that I could birth and deliver this project.

Angeles Arrien, Joan Borysenko, David Chamberlain, Bar bara Harper, Christiane Northrup, Michel Odent and Thoma

Contents

Foreword

More than a book, you hold in your hand an invitation. This wise and wonderful work invites you to sit under a great and spreading tree and learn with your heart how the world sings itself into being. It is filled with stories and practices that remind our spirit of the loving ways we can nurture each new life as it mysteriously joins us on earth, and ways we can nurture one another as well.

When I first heard the story that begins this book, I felt a longing to live in such an African village. I wanted to live in a world where each child, each person, is known and loved for her unique song.

We are born, as Wordsworth wrote, "trailing clouds of glory." Each child is a marvel. An old Hindu story tells of a baby in the womb singing, "Do not let me forget who I am." Then after birth the baby cries, "Oh I am forgetting already."

Unfortunately modern consumer society reflects this forgetting, and we live all too often in the absence of the sacred. Modern medicine and childbirth practices have frequently forgotten the soul. And how we raise the next generation, whether with soulless video and virtual daycare or loving community, will create the people of the world to be. This is a terribly urgent matter.

In *Welcoming The Soul of a Child*, Jill Hopkins offers us

an old treasure, a remembering of how to hear the song of the children born to us and of how to live with one another honoring the soul's song. Like a gardener she teaches us to prepare the soil of our hearts, to fertilize and nourish ourselves, and foster a ground of sacred respect and compassion within which our children will blossom.

Each child is a reflection of the divine, each birth an opportunity for us to again learn the great and only lesson of love. Through the heart's willing practices of meditation, prayers, sacred intention, and love songs, Jill Hopkins reminds us that we can heal and bless and honor life in each moment. We can learn again to live in this way.

May this book, and our devotion to our children, family, community, and the earth, bring blessings and connectedness to all that lives.

Jack Kornfield
Spiritrock Center
Woodacre, California 1998

Introduction

The seed of this book began to germinate the moment that I read a passage from Jack Kornfield's beautifully written book, *A Path with Heart*. He tells of a tribe of people in East Africa who recognize the birth date of a child prior to conception. For this tribe, the child is born the first time the child is a thought in its mother's mind. When she wishes to conceive a child, she goes out into the bush and sits alone under a tree. There she waits and listens until she hears the song of the child that she will give birth to. Conception occurs, in the eyes of these people, at the moment this song is heard. The mother then returns home and teaches the song to the father, so that while making love the child's spirit is called to them. The midwives and villagers are then taught the melody, so that during labor and at the moment of birth itself the child is welcomed into this world with his or her very own special song. This same song is sung during childhood illnesses, personal celebrations, initiations, and rites of passage. And at the end of one's life, loved ones gather around the deathbed to sing this song for the very last time.

I wept when I read those words then, and I weep when I read them now. Every single person who I have shared this story with is somehow moved. Why does this tribe's custom touch us so deeply? How is it that their unique story can resonate with so many people? Could it be that listening to this story gently calls forth our own soul?

I have discovered both in my work as a psychotherapist and on my own personal journey that most of us yearn, often painfully so, for this type of honoring. Our souls are crying out for meaningful connection. As the incoming baby of the African tribe is met by the villagers with a special song, we ache for our loved ones to welcome, love, and acknowledge us. We long for our own soul's song to be received, sung, and cherished.

When our world provided rituals and ceremonies that acknowledged the natural rhythms and cycles of the land and people, every activity was imbued with symbolic meaning. These practices fostered an appreciation of the subtle as well as the more dramatic changes that shaped and designed our lives. We were genuinely connected to all living things, and we were connected to our individual intuition and wisdom. Life was sacred. Now as we move through our days, weeks, and years faster than the speed of light, the loveliness of many magnificent moments goes unnoticed.

My intention is not to romanticize or mythologize the ways of the past or the customs and practices of indigenous cultures. To do so demeans the integrity of that which we admire. But what we can do is glean some wisdom from these ancient teachings and adapt that which we find fruitful into our lives in an intimate and personal way.

I also do not mean to belittle modern day advances. We can appreciate the unimaginable leaps humankind has made scientifically and technologically. From just about anywhere, with the push of a button, we can connect with one another via satellite, computer, fax, or cellular phone. Yet, paradoxically, it is this same technology that can directly contribute to our feelings of disconnection, isolation, and loneliness. We are in touch, but out of touch. Connecting electronically will never replace real human contact: skin to skin, heart to heart, soul to soul.

Long before the advent of a technological world, our society cultivated an affinity for "the pursuit"—be it of progress, wealth, land, or whatever. More currently, our latest trends forsake our links to more meaningful roots for the "perfect" career, the "perfect" relationship, the "perfect" body, and even having the "perfect" baby or child. The pursuit of perfection has become our search for the Holy Grail.

Even with the best of intentions, our earnest desire to be productive, responsible, and "good"—let alone survive—can leave us feeling frustrated, exhausted, and empty. Sexual, physical, and emotional abuse, violence, homelessness, drug addiction, poverty, and the irreparable damage we are inflicting upon our physical environment are only some of the manifestations of a disconnected and wounded world.

Nowhere do these patterns have a more profound and disturbing impact than on the birth and development of our children. We all want to give our children the best that we can give. But how can we expect to truly care for them if we are too busy, too distracted, and basically just too unconscious to care for ourselves and our world in a nurturing and responsible way? As a result of our absenteeism, not only physically, but emotionally and spiritually as well, we have created a society of unmothered and unfathered children. How can we possibly connect with our children when we don't have a clue how to connect with ourselves? We mirror back to them a soul-less globe.

Thomas Yeomans, a gifted psychologist, teacher, and author *(The Soul Wound)*, whose work has also inspired this book, describes this disconnection from ourselves and our lives that arises from not having our own souls honored and met. That pain manifests itself in our relationship to ourself, loved ones, and the world. Yeomans refers to this pain as a "soul wound."

We as a culture can no longer disguise, hide, or shield ourselves from the profound wounding that is taking place deep beneath the surface of our lives. It is from these depths that we cry out for meaningful connection—to reunite with the essence of our being—our soul.

This essence or true nature is what I believe to be the soul. It is that which embodies all of who we truly are. John Welwood talks about the soul in his book, *Love and Awakening,* ". . . as not something 'in' the body. Rather, it is a way of referring to what animates the body—our individual, embodied beingness, the living process that we are, with roots in the universal. It is, in Sri Aurobindo's words, 'a spark of the divine.' "

Welcoming The Soul of a Child is meant to offer ways in which we might awaken our innate capacity to recognize and honor our children as sacred beings with individual gifts. To welcome with open hearts and minds their "soul" self.

This is not a book about easy answers or quick how-to's, because there are none. However, it is my hope that we can begin to reacknowledge the sacredness of our lives, and most importantly, recognize the sacredness in our role as parent, teacher, and guide to our children. I would like to believe that somehow in this quest to see the holiness in our relationships, we might then begin to heal some of the disturbing trends that have severely injured us all.

Babies do not arrive with instruction manuals (although, you will hear stories in this book from people who will beg to differ). However, if a guidebook somehow magically appeared tucked in the belly buttons of our children upon their arrival, the opening page would insist that we, as their primary caretaker, must rediscover, reconnect, and celebrate our own lost soul. Whenever we do this for ourselves, it clears the way for us to truly see and hear our child's soul song. The writing of this book is a tribute to that wish.

My vision for *Welcoming The Soul of a Child* is to offer a

handbook—or you might say, a heartbook—of sorts, that invites the family and most particularly, mothers and fathers and other loved ones who have a strong presence in a child's life, to acknowledge, honor, and celebrate the souls of their children. But we need to take a vow to be solidly committed to our own growth mentally, emotionally, and spiritually. The purpose of this book is to guide you along that path, as well as provide invaluable resources for additional support. Whether you are carrying a child in your womb or carrying a child from someone else's arms into your own, such as in adoption or foster-parenting, I believe the basis of what I offer here can easily be adapted to anyone caring for a child. Whatever your family configuration or how you have come to cradle a child—what truly matters is the quality and manner in which we tend to and care for these exquisite incoming souls.

My experience as a hypnotherapist, working with literally hundreds of people, leaves no doubt in my mind that our prebirth, birth, and early years' experience have a huge influence on the unfolding of who we are as human beings. How we are welcomed, loved, respected, and cared for by those who have invited us here creates the sacred ground where we can root ourselves on this earthly plane; to sing our soul's song.

Studies and personal accounts consistently reflect that as a prenate, newborn, and child, we have a consciousness. Our children come into our bodies, our hearts, and our world awake, alert, and aware. They are magnificently seeded into this life, whole, complete—carrying their life's purpose. Acknowledging this, coupled with doing our own personal healing work, are the two greatest gifts that we can ever give to our children.

The African tribe in Kornfield's account seems to know this, as do many other tribal societies. But for a vast number of complex reasons, we as a modern culture seem to have forgotten or simply have chosen not to acknowledge this truth.

Ideally, a prerequisite for birthing a child would be to birth and heal the part of our own self that is wounded—or at least begin the journey to do so. And please know that it is never too late to heal our wounds. In fact, this exploration into our own wounds is the work of a lifetime. You can be assured it will not be an easy road to travel. However, it will be an adventure, one in which we will discover moments of truth and meaning, and where we can reconnect with our soul's song and gifts.

My hope is that *Welcoming The Soul of a Child* will inspire you to begin a lifelong commitment to genuinely value and love your children as they unfold and blossom throughout all of their lives. Becoming a parent is taking on a divine duty to protect, nurture, and guide. The divine gift given in return is the experience of the deepest and most profound love. As the tribe sings the individual's unique song, may we, too, find our own traditions and practices that welcome and embrace our children in a similarly personal, intimate, and respectful way.

It is said that our children are our most sacred temples. Let us go there now and listen as they sing their most unique and exquisite songs, so heart-filled, passionate, and pure.

> *The souls of pure teachers are arriving like rays of sunlight.*
>
> RUMI

Prelude

Welcoming the soul of a child is not a singular grand response to one biological event (momentous as it is!). Welcoming the soul of a child is a lifetime practice. Remember, the song that greets the baby from the East African tribe is one that is sung throughout that person's life.

The chapters that follow will focus on the time that envelops the experience of bringing a child into the world: from preparing to conceive to moving through the stages of conception, pregnancy, and birth. The final chapter will invite you to continue to view your relationship with your child as one that eternally unfolds, blossoms, and deepens throughout all of your life.

Being devoted to our own healing work can foster an awareness and the ability to see our children without filters tinted with our own unfulfilled expectations, unresolved fears, angers, and hurts. We can see them as the "pure teachers" that they are, "a spark of the divine," singing their soul's song as clear as a meditation bell! If we can see the opportunity to be a mother or father as the gift that it truly is and to use this gift as impetus for our own personal healing, just imagine the boundless value to all.

> ... and the more souls who resonate together,
> the greater the intensity of their love, and,
> mirror-like, each soul reflects the other.

DANTE

Who This Book Is For

Welcoming The Soul of a Child is written primarily for individuals who are anywhere in the stages of birthing a child— from exploring the possibility of becoming a parent (biologically or through adoption), to trying to conceive, to being pregnant and preparing for birth. It is also written for parents who might have already adopted or given birth to a child. And although the book directs much of the material to the parent, many of the exercises will be supportive and worthwhile to anyone who is dedicated to their healing work and who cares passionately for children.

How to Use the Book

Reading this book before you conceive a baby is ideal. However, the essence of the material, including a good number of the exercises and rituals, can be helpful at any time during your life's journey.

In other words, although there are some exercises and rituals that are stage specific *(Creating a Birth Plan, Visualizations for Labor and Birth*, etc.) there are many that can be adapted for other purposes besides childbearing *(Accessing Our Inner Wisdom, Creating a Sacred Space, Healing Our Losses*, etc.).

So although you might be physically paralleling the stages highlighted in each chapter (conception, pregnancy . . .), there are many skills, exercises, and rituals that are not chronologically focused. Use the *Index* in the back of the book to find

Exercises, Rituals, Ceremonies, and Celebrations according to topic.

Elements of the Book

Cultivating Skills (such as *Listening, Being Present,* or *Lovingkindness*) teaches and reenforces essential ingredients for being more present in our lives, while integrating and harmonizing the fragmented and disconnected aspects of ourselves. Most of the skills correspond to a specific *Exercise* and/or *Ritual,* where you are given opportunities to practice using that particular skill. In fact, all of the *exercises* are meant to ground, anchor, and put into action what we are learning in our minds. *Stories: Traditional and Personal,* share intimate experiences, while honoring the universal pains and joys of birthing a child. They inspire, teach, and remind us just how deeply connected we all are. *Rituals, Ceremonies, and Celebrations* offer a way to honor the sacred passages in your life while further deepening your healing. They also give opportunities to express appreciation and gratitude for the gifts given to you on your life's journey.

At the back of the book I have provided *Recomended Reading, Resources* (including helpful organizations and videos pertaining to childbirth) and an *Index,* which arranges the *Exercises, Rituals, Ceremonies, and Celebrations* by category.

Please note: whenever you come to an exercise or ritual, read through it first and see if you resonate with it. It may be an experience that you choose to do now, or at a later time, or not at all. As mentioned previously, the exercises, rituals, ceremonies, and celebrations are not necessarily chronological, nor are they all applicable to everyone. They are meant to provide a reservoir of experiences to choose from, which may be helpful to you on your healing adventure. When you are ready to do any of them, read through them and then write brief notes, make a simple outline, or record it on an audio cassette to follow. You can also have your birth partner or a friend read the words and lead you through the process.

All of the elements offered here are given with the hope that they will encourage, support, and inspire you to adapt them as your own. And most importantly, although this is sacred stuff—have fun. Remember, children love to play!

. . . then the babe knew that it wouldn't be long now, and the moon shone a little brighter, for, although many people think that the moon gets its light from reflection, it is love which is the source of all light. And the baby laughed.

SHERRIL JAFFE
The Baby Laughs

1

Calling Forth the Child
PRE-CONCEPTION

I've never been a great sleeper. There have been certain times in my life, however, when surrendering to nocturnal slumber was effortless. It was during one of those times, several years ago, that I experienced the most curious thing.

On a breezy and rainy spring night, I found myself gently stirred from a deep and lovely sleep by something that seemed even lovelier. It was a woman's voice, humming melodically. At first, I was sure that I was dreaming. But my eyes were open. When I was awake enough, I sat up to see if I could see my visitor. Oddly enough, I was not frightened. (You must understand that although I have been known to be extremely intuitive at times, I have never seen any unmanifested beings at the foot of my bed. I much prefer visiting over a cup of tea or a latte.) The moment that I sat up, though, the humming abruptly stopped. Although I can't be sure how long I had been serenaded, the episode probably lasted less than a minute.

Following the visit, I couldn't go back to sleep. Interestingly enough, I didn't feel disturbed by the woman's presence—just intrigued and puzzled. Lying in bed, wondering about all of this, I noticed a willow tree outside my bedroom window. Funny how I had never really seen it before. As the wind tenderly rocked the upper branches back and forth, I observed how intertwining vines and twigs created a goddesslike shape centered right in the heart of the tree. Just before being lulled back into sleep, I realized the most amazing thing! Just as the African woman listens beneath the tree for the song of the child she will conceive, I, too, had been whispered a song. A song that would become the essence of this book.

It has always felt like *Welcoming The Soul Of A Child* has had a soul. From the very beginning it felt like I was birthing a child. So whether the song that I heard on that rainy spring night was that of the soul of this book, of my own soul, or a harmony of the two, it is my wish that its melody will emanate through these words and somehow inspire you to listen for your child's and your own soul's song.

PREPARING THE GARDEN

To honor the "calling forth of the child," this chapter will focus on the necessity of creating a welcoming environment for the incoming spirit even before conception. I like to think of it as preparing the garden before we seed.

Before planting the seeds in any garden, it is essential to envision what we wish to create and why. We then need to dig into the ground and remove the weeds, roots, and rocks that may be found there—all of which would surely inhibit the sprouting of new life.

In just the same way, as we prepare for the conception and ultimate birth of our child, we, too, must first contemplate, imagine, and give considerable thought to why we wish to be a parent. It is part of methodically and consciously preparing the soil in which a child can ultimately seed and grow. Just as in digging the garden, this can be very hard work. Yet, the blood, sweat, and tears of our labor brings forth a healthier body, mind, and heart—primary ingredients for creating a safe and luxurious environment for the budding of new life.

As we prepare the garden for planting the seeds, or conceiving a baby, let's consider the body, mind, heart, and soul dimensions of this process.

Body

Whether you are female or male, strengthening your body with nourishing, wholesome foods is imperative. If you are unsure how to begin a healthier regimen, talk to your doctor, a naturopath, nutritionist, or midwife. Regular exercise is important as well. Besides helping you to feel better about the way your body looks, your heart, lungs, and blood will function much more efficiently. Sufficient sleep, or creating more quiet or downtime, provides the opportunity for your mind, body, and heart to restore and rejuvenate itself. All of these things contribute to an overall sense of well-being, making you a vibrant vessel for new life. Remember, if you don't feel you know how to incorporate this way of being in your daily life or you just need support, talk to a professional who specializes in health and fitness. Or spend time with friends who are already involved in taking good care of themselves.

Just as the garden's fertile ground promotes germination, a strong and healthy body provides the ideal setting for conception and the development of a healthy baby. And believe me, being fit now will not only help you during the physical birth, but also with meeting the rigorous demands of parenting down the road, when physical and mental fatigue are a given!

You also might consider the importance of your surroundings. Our physical home can definitely reflect our inner home. You might give some thought to how your habitat reflects your state of mind, physical health, self-esteem, relationships, and unresolved and unfinished business.

This is an ideal time to clean attics, closets, and drawers, and to paint, remodel, or repair whatever needs attending to. In addition to marveling at our cleaner and more organized abode, we will feel more refreshed and rejuvenated as the "cleaning up" magically becomes a metaphor in action. Living in this world fraught with social and cultural demands and pressures, quality time at home and working on improving our overall health and wellness can serve as a perfect healing remedy.

Create time and space for preparing "the nest." Whether you restore the living space where you now live or decide to move to a new one, begin to fill it with qualities of warmth, security, wellness, and love.

Mind

It is also invaluable and crucial to look at any thought or behavioral patterns that might be improved. I can not stress this enough. Whatever distracts and clouds us from being truthful and present with ourselves, will severely restrict our capacity to be available to our children. In addition to the exercises offered throughout the book, which are meant to support your desire and intention to be as healthy and conscious as you can, you may find other forms of healing practices helpful (e.g., psychotherapy, hypnotherapy, movement therapy, body work, acupuncture, meditation, yoga, biofeedback, tai chi, aikido, Qi gong, etc.). Any healing modality that you resonate with can only facilitate more self-knowledge and awareness—the context or foundation which allows us to better understand and see ourselves and our children.

> ... *when the mind is clear you can see all the way to the heart.*
>
> —STEPHEN LEVINE

Clearing the mind is a way to recognize the vastness of our being. When we learn how to have more compassion for who we are, we minimize the risk of setting up injuring expectations for our children that arise solely from our own unmet needs and disowned parts of ourselves.

Investigating our fear, anger, resentments, and other forms of wounding leads us deeper into our pain, which contains a lifetime of grief and suffering. And if we dare to journey further, it is where we might touch the unfathomable rawness and tenderness of our soul wound. Through the process of digging in the soil and uprooting the unconscious self-destructive patterns, we create more space in the garden and in our hearts for the potential of new life—ours and our child's. The pain, once excruciating, becomes the bridge leading us back to our own home—to our own true essence where we discover our soul's gifts.

Heart

We armor our hearts (usually unconsciously) as a result of enduring the soul wound. Paradoxically, the armor that attempts to shield and distance us from pain is the same armor that blocks us from the experience of love and happiness. As we go deeper into our healing process, we discover that we can't touch into any authentic feelings unless we work through the pain. Puddle-jumping unresolved issues or playing spiritual leapfrog will not bring us any closer to our truth or our genuine self. In fact, it will only keep us at a greater distance. Connecting to, remembering, and working toward healing the pain, illuminates and honors more of who we truly are. It is the pain that guides us back onto our soul's path.

As we work diligently to clear the mind, care for the physical body, and nurture our spirit, the heart begins to soften and open naturally. Actually, the heart always remains open, much like the sun eternally shines. What we are actually doing is dislodging the hard-crusted mantel that blocks the heart from loving. This becomes some of our deepest inner work. A practice of lovingkindness and compassion eases, softens, and dissolves this hardened part of ourself. This is precious work.

You see, if we are unable to love or appreciate ourselves (and I don't mean this in the narcissistic way—narcissism, in the simplest of terms, is an overcompensation or defensive reaction to not feeling loved or valued) it will be extremely difficult for us to allow our children to express their love to us. Rather than openly receiving their gifts of love, we will purposefully or inadvertently push them away. Any false belief about ourselves, regarding our lack of worth or lack of lovableness, will make us resist, reject, run and hide from the very thing that we long for. Of course, this is usually all unconscious, which makes it even more disturbing. With this in mind we have to wonder what we are teaching our children about love and loving and their own lovableness. When we reject (consciously or unconsciously) that which is so natural and intrinsic to who they are, it is as though we are taking a razor-sharp blade and slowly carving out the makings of their soul wound.

This is why our inner work is of paramount importance— and why it is the work of a lifetime. We need to learn how to embrace the disowned and fragmented parts of ourselves with tenderness and compassion, and to understand the origins of our own wounds and their effect on our relationships. Only then can we open our arms and hearts to the totality of our child. This includes the wounded child that lives within all of us, as well as our future biological or adopted child. The commitment to our own personal and spiritual growth begins to transform our soul wound into sweet nectar; nectar that with a sense of delight and joy nurtures and nourishes our child's soul-self, as well as our own.

> *Let us be grateful to people who make us happy;*
> *they are the charming gardeners who make our*
> *souls blossom.*
>
> —MARCEL PROUST

All in all, we can create the most idyllic outward conditions to grow whatever we want, yet if there is not the passionate heartfelt caring and commitment to accompany the action, the hope for vibrant, vital, and spirited life is diminished significantly. If our children are nourished, guided, protected, and cared for with utmost tenderness and conscious awareness, we will witness their unfolding petal by petal, blossoming into their most ravishing beauty.

CULTIVATING SKILLS

Cultivating and practicing the following skills foster more awareness and strengthen and deepen our relationship to our self, our lives, and to our loved ones. Developing these skills, especially *Soul Glimpses,* provide the path home where we can hear our own soul singing.

Being Present

There are some wonderful books written on the subject of *Being Present* or what is also known as Mindfulness (see *Recommended Reading*). Very simply, *Being Present* is cultivating the practice of moment to moment awareness so that we might experience our life more fully and with a greater sense of meaning and purpose. So often, our thoughts are lost in the past or racing into the future. Consequently, we miss the preciousness of the now. And in the context of being a mother or father, that means we will often miss seeing the inner beauty and potential that lives within our child.

Thich Nhat Hanh, a Buddhist monk, meditation teacher, and poet, exquisitely teaches about the importance of mindfulness or being present in his book, *The Art of Mindful Living*. He talks about how the moon, which wishes to reflect its beautiful light onto a pond, is unable to do so if the pond is not still and calm. If the pond's water is moving, the moon's reflection will be a disturbing distortion of its pure splendor.

It is a poignant metaphor that describes the importance of practicing *Being Present*. It also conveys how our state of being can directly affect how our child perceives herself. As children develop physically, psychologically, and spiritually, they look to us to mirror back to them their true beauty. If our pond or our state of being is cloudy, restless, and agitated, our child will look into our eyes and misread who she truly is.

The value of cultivating the skill of *Being Present* is multifold—from helping us restore ourselves to a more balanced and calm state, to bringing more wisdom, understanding, and awareness into our daily living. This is most especially true in our relationship to our child.

Deep Breathing, Meditation, Listening and incorporating ritual into our life are some of the ways in which we can begin to sharpen our skills of being more present.

> *There is only one place where love can be found, where intimacy and awakening can be found, and that is in the present. When we live in our thoughts of the past and future, everything seems distant, hurried and unfulfilled. The only place we can genuinely love a tree, the sky, a child, or our lover is in the here and now.*
>
> —Jack Kornfield

Soul Glimpses

Throughout the book, I encourage you to listen for your own soul's song. One way that you might begin to get in touch with your song is to become keenly aware of what profoundly moves you in the course of the day. This will be a challenge, given the frenetic pace of our lives. Yet, it is a great opportunity to practice Mindfulness and *Being Present*. It is also a golden way to get a glimpse of our soul.

Because if we are paying attention, we just might find one instance where something catches our eye. We become captivated and enchanted—we literally stop—for that moment. A marker may be the way our breathing changes from rapid and shallow to slow and even. We may even experience a magical sense of calm and peace. This moment will go unnoticed and vanish in the blink of an eye, unless we allow ourselves the luxury to be fully in it. This noticing may be found in any moment; ones that feel dynamic and dramatic or (where I have generally discovered them) in the simple and ordinary. It is where we discover a hint of our soul expressing itself.

The following exercise is one where your soul's passions may reveal themselves to you. The questions come from a Thomas Yeomans workshop on Spiritual Psychology.

Sitting comfortably in a special place, and after centering yourself with deep breathing, ask yourself the following questions. This can be a meditation and/or you can write the answers down. It is important to give yourself all the time you need, yet the first responses are the ones that are usually the most authentic.

> *What troubles me most about the world is* . . . .
> *What I love most about the world is* . . . .

How does your life reflect and/or actively express these strong feelings? How might you channel these passions in a way that feels genuine and fulfilling? Write your thoughts in a journal (see *Creative Journaling*) and, if you wish, share them with your partner.

Self-Nurturing

When you think of self-nurturing, think of filling a cup, a goblet, or a well with the purest and most refreshing water. Self-nurturing, not to be confused with self-absorption, is a practice of nourishing and replenishing yourself in a healthy way—of filling your cup. When our cup is empty, we have nothing to sustain ourself, let alone give to those we love. When our cup is full, the overflow goes to those we care about, as well as keeping us healthy and strong. Cultivating a Self-nurturing Practice is always important. It is especially beneficial to you as you prepare for and enter into parenthood. We are more refreshed, healthy, and clear when we are taking good care of ourselves. Just as the pure water overflows from a full cup, so does the water that is toxic or polluted. What is it that we wish to feed our baby and child?

To begin a self-nurturing practice, simply sit down and write out all of the things that help to make you feel nourished; free associate. Highlight ten of these things and rank them according to their importance. Then figure out a way to incorporate the first three into your daily or weekly life. See if you can add one or two more as a monthly—or once every three months—self-nurturing activity. (In view of our busy lives, leaving your schedule open on a particular afternoon can be extremely nourishing and serve as self-nurturing time! A self-nurturing practice is not about complicating your life, but rather simplifying it).

Write these nurturing ideas on a piece of paper. Put the note on a windowsill, up on your refrigerator door, or on your bathroom mirror. Let it be a reminder to take good care of yourself. If you have to, schedule this nurturing time in your datebook and do not accept any cancellations!

Nourishing and Strengthening Our Relationship

A relationship is a dynamic and living thing. And just like anything that is alive, it needs to be tenderly nurtured. Devoting time and energy to the relationship with our partner will be vitally important not only to ourselves, but to our child.

Cultivating this practice will be reenforced by doing our own healing work, learning good communication skills, and being dedicated to the relationship's growth. I have recommended excellent books on this theme. However, as we pass through the threshold of becoming a mother or father to our baby and child, we have the opportunity to go even further into our relationship. The exercises and rituals for the couple's relationship offer many possibilities for creating a more intimate and compassionate connection to one another, while exploring and discovering deeper truths.

Exploring Your Resistance

When doing your personal and relationship work, you may feel, from time to time, resistant to doing an exercise, practicing a skill, or even participating in a celebration. You may become numb, sleepy, agitated, or annoyed. This is to be expected, as our current self-image/identity typically does not like to be challenged or threatened. We much prefer the comfort and safety of the familiar. Yet there is a powerful part of our personality that has developed solely in response to or in defense against a world that we perceive as not welcoming and safe. For protection we end up creating masks to hide behind. Without self-awareness and understanding, it is very difficult to know whether or not we are living our life genuinely or authentically. The more we hide, the more we become disconnected from our true self and our soul's song.

Disguised since childhood,
haphazardly assembled
from voices and fears and little pleasures,
We come of age as masks
Our true face never speaks
—RAINER MARIA RILKE

Yet as you begin your inner work and discover insights, make connections, and touch into your genuine self, you will realize that it takes a lot less energy to be with yourself truthfully and authentically than to maintain your defenses. And as you utilize the skills that you are learning and begin to feel safer, you can begin to ease up on the fierce intensity with which you hold on to the mask.

Our commitment and promise (to ourself and to our children) to grow and heal, requires great courage. Through imagery, writing, movement, and drawing, we can acquaint ourselves with the one holding up the mask. Through the technique of *dialoguing* we can connect with the part of our being who is hiding, terrified and lost. Practicing the tools that we are learning, either on our own and/or with a healing professional, can help us transform the resistance, fear, sorrow, and sometimes terror into something much more useful and powerful. We can use it as a messenger from our deepest and darkest self. It is here that we can begin to hear the voice . . . the song of the soul.

Although we might like to think of love only in terms
of the light it brings into our life, if we are not
also willing to confront the darkness that this light
reveals, our soul will never ripen or evolve.
—JOHN WELWOOD

Creative Journaling

Creative Journaling is a wonderful practice that provides an intimate, sacred place for expressing our thoughts and feelings. All you need are pens, paper, and a little quiet time. You can either purchase a journal from a bookstore or make your own by putting loose paper in a three-ring notebook. I like to write in one of those black leather sketchbooks that you can find in various sizes at art supply stores. You can either structure a specific time to write, or carry your journal with you, so that you might jot down thoughts when you feel moved to do so. You can also use the journal for doing exercises in this book or any other inner and couple's work that you might be engaged in. In *The Couple's Comfort Book,* Jennifer Louden suggests keeping a couple's journal, where romantic notes, dreams, feelings, and even thoughts on conflicting issues are written and shared with one another. Writing in your journal can enhance your growth by providing a venue to process what you are learning, or to illuminate and celebrate your spiritual growth. Record your own thoughts, drawings, inner journey exercises, nondominant hand exercises, excerpts from inspiring poetry and prose, song lyrics, photographs, dreams, fantasies, and even letters to your unborn child; these are just some of the ways that your journal can serve as a sacred recording of your expanding consciousness. It may even provide a sacred place for you to connect with your child.

Dialoguing

In both my personal and professional work, I have found the technique of *dialoguing* extraordinarily effective. It's a powerful way to access our inner wisdom, while transforming what appears as an obstacle into something healing.

We can dialogue with everything and anything that is in need of deeper understanding and compassion. We can dialogue with our physical pains, fears, grief, and even with our unborn child.

When working with clients and doing my own personal work, I have found visual imagery one of the most effective ways of utilizing this technique. However, you can dialogue through drawing, writing, body movement, and even using your dreams. *Dialoguing* is a process where, by literally having a conversation with a part of yourself, you are able to access messages that are not usually transmitted in ordinary states of consciousness.

EXERCISES

These exercises support self-growth and awareness through the practice of quieting oneself and going within *(meditation, deep breathing, creating a sacred space)*. For it is in stillness that we can better access our own inner wisdom and even hear our own soul's song. The exercises for couples *(couple's sanctuary, contemplating parenthood, mandorla exercises)* guide us on the path of true intimacy, including exploring our feelings about becoming a mother or father.

Creating A Sacred Space

Sacred space can be found anywhere. It is a special place in your home where you can meditate, practice deep breathing exercises, listen to music, read, write, draw, or just rest in silence. It can be a favorite chair, porch swing, garden bench, a cushion on the floor—it's anywhere that is private, quiet, comfortable, and safe.

A *sacred space* can be simple and austere, or you can embellish it with personal and intimate objects—candles, books, photographs, artwork, seashells, polished stones, a quilt, or flowers—whatever helps to invoke a sense of well-being.

My sacred space consists of a lovely, velvety, wine-colored sofa surrounded by cherished photographs and books, candles, and a basket full of pine cones, hawk feathers and stones (all of the things that, as a family, we have collected on our nature walks). It's where I retreat to read, meditate, write in my journal, and even write some of these pages.

Your *sacred space* will be the perfect environment to do many of the rituals, ceremonies, and exercises that are suggested throughout this book. Overall, it is a safe and peaceful place where you can practice caring for yourself in a loving and respectful way during all of the phases of birthing a child.

As you design this space, be imaginative. Let your heart guide and direct you. Allow your sacred space to emanate your very own soul's song. You can bless this place daily or create a special ritual of blessing. (See *Blessing the Sacred Place Ritual*)

Open Heart Meditation

In your *sacred space,* light a candle, sit quietly, and place your right hand on the center of your chest. Take a deep breath. Connect to your breath. Feel the pulsing of your heart. Allow the warmth of your hand to soothe this part of your body. Notice the sensations. Breathe slowly and gently. Feel or visualize your heart softening and opening. Breathe in and breathe out. Imagine holding or seeing a baby, or any other person or image that evokes a feeling of love in your heart's center. Notice the sensations and thoughts that arise. Breathe in warmth and love. Breathe out any discomfort or tightness that you might feel in your chest or anywhere else in your body. Breathe in. Breathe out. Imagine your heart softening and opening. Feel any discomfort or tightness easing. Feel the warmth of your hand continuing to soothe your heart center. This is a perfect time to also ask yourself if there is anything that you need to know at this particular time. Listen for your response. Breathe in. Breathe out. Feel the warmth moving through all of your body. Feel your mind opening and expanding. Breathe in. Breathe out. Allow yourself all of the time that you need.

This meditation can be a wonderful beginning for any exercise, ritual or ceremony, particularly when you add a prayer or blessing. It can also be utilized as an invaluable tool when experiencing a particular challenge or any overwhelming feelings.

Deep Breathing

It seems rather ironic that we need to be reminded how to do something that is most essential and natural to our survival. But I suppose our style of breathing reflects how we move in our lives—from rapid to shallow to forgetting to breathe at all!

If you want to learn more about developing a deep breathing practice see *Recommended Reading*. There are wonderful books and tapes available for this purpose. Since deep breathing is integral to yoga, Qi gong, stretching and relaxation exercises, meditation etc., you might consider enrolling in some classes.

A simple introduction to deep breathing is to first sit comfortably with your spine erect. Close your eyes and bring your awareness to your breath. Focus on taking in a nice full and deep breath. Hold it to the count of four. Now breathe out evenly on the count of four. Repeat this three or four times. Then follow your breath. Allow it to find its own natural rhythm. Keep focusing on the breath. You can say to yourself, "I'm breathing in ease and relaxation. I'm breathing out tightness, discomfort. Breathing in. Breathing out." When you find your mind wandering off or becoming distracted, simply remind yourself to focus once again on the breath. "Breathing in that which comes in. Breathing out that which goes out. So easy and effortless. Just noticing. Nothing to do or know . . . merely breathing in and breathing out." When your session is coming to an end, inhale one deep breath to the count of four. Exhale slowly to the count of four.

Practice at least five minutes daily in your *sacred space*. Use waiting in any line (such as at the post office or the market) or while sitting at a stop light when in your car, as bonus time to strengthen this invaluable skill. In addition to doing the breathing exercise, I like to bring my right palm to my chest over my heart (see *Open Heart Meditation*). Simply bringing my hand to this part of my body, and sometimes moving it in a circular fashion, triggers a spontaneous calming effect. As you cultivate this deep breathing skill, you will find your breath a useful tool for centering and grounding yourself in a myriad of situations.

Meditation

There are as many ways to meditate as there are ways to sit and breathe. I've taught meditation for a number of years, and always encourage people to discover and create their own personal practice. Teachers, retreats, books, and tapes can be instructive and inspiring, but ultimately, your daily practice will offer the richest experiences. All that you need is a time (when you will not be interrupted), a quiet place (you may find your *sacred space* ideal) and your willingness to sit, breathe, and listen. Either read and record the following guided meditation on an audio cassette (to listen to when you wish to practice) or read through the words to get the essence of the practice and then adapt them in your own personal and unique way.

Begin your practice by sitting on the floor, a cushion, couch, or chair. Sit comfortably with your spine erect. Take a moment to adjust your body. Close your eyes if you wish. Remind yourself that you need not be anywhere else but right here. Then, simply follow the rhythm of your breath. Breathe in and breathe out. Follow the natural rhythm of your breath. There is no need to push or force. . . .merely allowing. Allowing your breath to do what it knows to do. Breathing in and breathing out. Breathing so easily and effortlessly. Notice any sensations that arise. Just noticing. Allow yourself to feel the sensations. Breathe through them slowly and evenly. Breathing in and breathing out. Notice any holding or tightness. Breathe into that place—especially there. Feel the breath easing away the holding or tightness. The breath feels so soothing and calming. Feel the breath moving in and then moving out. Noticing the thoughts of the mind coming and then going. Breathe through them, as well. Allowing the breath to come in and then allowing the breath to go out. The breath flows so easily and effortlessly. Resting in the breath, now. Allowing yourself now, to breathe in the quiet . . . into the silence. (Give yourself several minutes of quiet). Now gently return to the breath. Breathing in. Breathing out. Allowing the breath to slowly and easily carry you into a more wakeful state. When opening your eyes you will feel energized, awake, yet rested and peaceful. Take your time. Whenever you are ready—open your eyes.

There are many variations of this particular meditation. It is only one way to begin a practice. Refer to *Recommended Reading* for further and more in-depth study.

Couple's Sanctuary

A couple's sanctuary is *sacred space* for two. The *couple's sanctuary* is a physical place that is exclusively designed for the two of you. It can be inside or outside the home. It can be one specific place, such as a favorite little nook in your bedroom, a favorite couch, a front porch swing, a certain park bench, or a hot tub. My husband and I have had our greatest talks in a small, claw-footed, antique bathtub. Somehow, turning off the artificial lights, lighting candles, and pouring our bodies into the hot water, along with the bubbles and essential oils, provides the perfect intimate setting for our sacred sharing. It could be a place co-created in the moment, using whatever is available (cushions, a special place that you find on a walk, sitting in front of a fire). The most important element, however, is bringing to this place a quality of honoring your relationship and each other in a respectful and sacred way.

Wherever your sanctuary is, it's imperative that both partners feel safe, comfortable, and assured that they will not be interrupted (you may need to take extra measures for this one—turn off the phones, put a please-do-not-disturb sign on the door, select your time wisely, etc.). Ideally it is an environment where you can just be together and, if you wish, a place to practice some of the suggested exercises.

The *couple's sanctuary* is a place where you can cuddle, hold each other, give each other a massage, write in your journal, read, meditate together, and more. It may be helpful to agree upon certain rules for this place. For example, have a plan for how you might respond if intense emotions are triggered during an exercise. It is absolutely critical that this place remains safe. If emotions are accelerating and you find yourself blaming and judging each other, consider taking a break (take a walk, get a glass of water, sit alone quietly). But always do this with the intention that you will return and bring some sense of closure to the session. When you come back together, restate the purpose of the exercise. It doesn't necessarily take the intensity away, but can help you refocus and ground the work, as well as yourselves. If what is coming up feels particularly challenging, you might consider working with a healing professional.

The *couple's sanctuary* is a sacred place. In time, just entering into it should make you and your partner feel honored, nourished, and strengthened.

Contemplating Parenthood
(A Couple's Exercise)

Part of nourishing and strengthening our relationship with our partner is to open up a dialogue about how we see ourselves, individually and as a couple. This dialogue offers an opportunity to explore our strengths, as well as the areas in the relationship that need our attention. This assessment is not only helpful in better understanding and improving your relationship, but allows for more clarity and truthfulness when you begin to explore the idea of birthing a child together. Take a walk, wake up at sunrise, or sit together in the *couple's sanctuary* and contemplate the following questions. Either write the answers separately in your personal journals and then share them with each other, or discuss aloud your responses.

- What are our individual and collective strengths?
- What are our individual and collective weaknesses?
- How do we respond to everyday demands and pressures?
- What can we do individually and together to improve those responses? (e.g., relaxation training, deep breathing, cultivating a self-nurturing practice, setting clearer boundaries)
- What are our honest feelings about becoming parents? (Include your fears).
- How might our individual and collective strengths and weaknesses impact becoming a parent?
- What might we learn individually and together as a couple to strengthen our relationship? What issues need to be addressed? (You might consider exploring these questions in one-on-one counseling and/or couple's therapy, a relationship workshop, or retreat)
- Why do you want to become a mother or father?
- What do you imagine you will offer your child(ren)?
- What do you imagine your child(ren) will teach you?

Dialoguing With Our Resistance

In your *sacred space* or any place that is safe and quiet, center yourself with conscious breathing. Allow your breath to bring you fully into the moment. Become aware of the chair, floor, or cushion beneath you as that surface holds and supports your body. Remind yourself that there isn't any other place to be other than right here. Focus on breathing in and breathing out. Breathe in and out slowly and evenly until you feel relaxed and calm. Now invite "the resistance" to appear, however it wishes to be known. You may see visual images, hear sounds or words within, or simply experience body sensations. You can even ask, "Does this resistance reside anywhere in my body?" If so, ask where. Pay close attention to how your body is responding. (You might notice tightness in the throat, achiness in your lower back, burning sensations in your shoulders, etc.) As you continue to invite the resistance to present itself to you, keep noticing what emerges, whether it is from the body or mind.

At some point, ask the resistance what it wants you to know. What has it come to communicate to you? It may be useful to ask it to convey its message to you in words. You can keep dialoguing back and forth as long as needed. If for any reason you come to a stuck place, or you are feeling numb, blank, etc. (just other forms of resistance), dialogue with the stuck place, numbness, etc. Ultimately, you can dialogue with anything that spontaneously emerges in the exercise. Continue to dialogue until you receive a message that you understand. You can then ask, "What is it that I need to know or do to help me heal?" Notice if the imagery or sensations change. Write or draw what you learn in your journal.

Mandorla Exercise

The mandorla is a powerful symbol that comes from medieval Christianity. It is found in artwork and in cathedrals throughout Europe, often depicting the opposing forces of heaven and earth. You can see the almond-shaped mandorla symbol when two circles overlap. (In mathematics, this symbol is called a Venn diagram). (See Diagram A—page 23.)

What is powerful about the symbol is how it synergizes two opposing perspectives. It provides a tool for bridging and healing polarized, either/or thinking, which is devastating to any relationship—be it a relationship to yourself, to your partner, your child, or to the world.

In your *sacred space* or in the *couple's sanctuary*, draw five mandorla symbols; two for yourself, two for your partner, and one for the relationship.

First, do the exercise individually. Close your eyes and think of an issue that you are currently challenged by. For example, in the right circle write words that describe what you think of as "positives" about becoming a parent (sharing your love, feeling connected, creating a family). In the left circle write words that describe your opposing or "negative" thoughts and feelings (fearful of perpetuating unhealthy family patterns, losing your freedom). (See Diagram B—page 23.)

Now see if you can acknowledge that you hold both views, that in fact, for you each view has its truth. In honoring the validity in each, see if you can find what might lie within the core of the two. A hint here is to look at the opposing view and see if you can find the value in it. For example, you might see how fear motivates us to be cautious and discerning. You can write those words in the almond-shaped section. Then what words might you use to further describe your desire to share love and create a family? Perhaps you associate this with the qualities of commitment and devotion. Write those words in the almond-shaped segment of the diagram, too. Now reflect on the synergy of the two conflicting poles and create a healing statement, e.g., "I approach becoming a parent and creating a family with loving devotion, commitment, and discernment." Write this statement in your journal and/or write it out on a

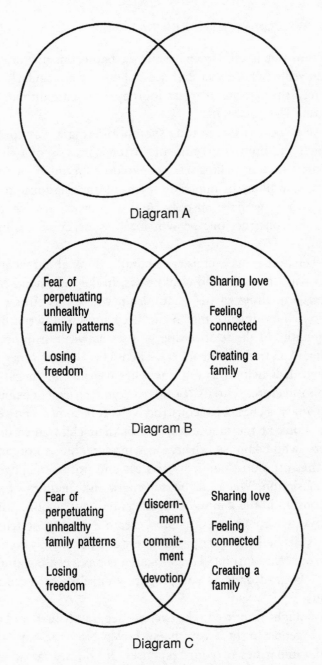

Diagram A

Diagram B

Diagram C

Healing statement: I approach becoming a parent with commitment, loving devotion, and discernment.

card and put it up somewhere (e.g., bathroom mirror, on a windowsill), where you can see it and say it regularly as a healing affirmation for your journey into parenthood. (See Diagram C—page 23.)

The mandorla is a healing symbol offering a way to work through the limitations and often the paralysis of either/or thinking. In our willingness to explore our inner opposing forces, as well as the opposing forces in our relationship with our partner, we have an opportunity to transform what can block and obstruct our growth into a synergy of healing in action.

When doing this exercise as a couple, think about what you see as your strengths and weaknesses. In the right-hand circle, write the qualities of the relationship you see as strong (e.g. loyalty, commitment) and in the left-hand circle write down the qualities of the relationship you see as weak or in need of healing (e.g., unresolved anger). Then reflect on the synergy of the two. It is helpful to reframe what we call the "negative," or opposing force, into its "positive" counterpart. For example, when anger is channeled constructively, it becomes a powerful force. Look at the mothers who lost their children to drunk drivers, who channeled their anger into creating an organization that promotes public awareness and positive changes in our legislation. Write all the adjectives and qualities of your relationship in the almond-shaped center (e.g., action, power, loyalty, and commitment). Now create a healing statement, such as "Together we are passionately and powerfully committed to our relationship." Use the statement as a healing affirmation to be read daily as you prepare yourselves for becoming parents.

You might want to do the exercise separately first, and then come together to share your perspectives. Note the similarities and dissimilarities of your responses. If you are far apart in your responses, talk about that and try again, or agree together on at least one or two of the qualities (both strong and weak).

Then create a synergy healing statement together. (See the *Couple's Healing Ritual* for an idea on how to take this exercise and adapt it for a sacred ceremony).

Weeding the Garden

This can be a delightfully freeing exercise. It is a metaphor in action for releasing and letting go of that which is no longer useful in our life. Think of doing this exercise when you are uprooting behavioral and emotional patterns that are hurtful to yourself and/or others. (e.g., blame, unresolved anger and resentments, self-loathing, compulsive behavior).

Write down what you wish to let go of on scrap pieces of paper or in the form of a letter. Once written, crumble the paper up into a ball or tear it into little pieces and then throw it all away into the trash. Burning the pieces of paper in a fireplace is also an excellent way of "letting go."

You can also weed a garden literally. As you pull up each weed, give it a name. When you are ready to discard the weeds, make a statement or affirmation of what you are digging up and releasing ("I willingly free myself of . . ."). When this is done, plant new seeds, tend to the ones already planted, or bed your garden down for the winter. And just as rotting and decaying plants make rich organic compost—one of the healthiest and most natural ways to promote a garden's growth—may we, too, find ways to utilize our own decomposing and spoiled parts, as minerals and nutrients for vibrant new life.

Your Birth Story

This is an ideal time to find out about your own birth. Ask your mother to tell you everything that she remembers about conceiving you, her pregnancy, and your birth. If your mother isn't alive or accessible, talk to other family members who might be able to share what they know. Or you can always write to the hospital where you were born and ask for your birth records (hospital birth records may indicate drugs used, if you were induced, if you were a surviving twin, or any complications that may have occurred with your birth). This exercise can be extremely helpful in understanding the manner in which we were or were not welcomed into the world. The physical and psychological wounding that we may have experienced (e.g., a difficult birth, not being wanted or not being the "right" gender, being abandoned, etc.) can directly affect the way in which we welcome our baby. Working toward healing this type of wounding begins by gathering information about our birth. Some of the questions that you might ask are:

Conception

- What were the circumstances of my conception? Was I planned and wanted, or was I a surprise? Was there ambivalence about my coming? Were there thoughts or attempts to abort me?
- Had there been any previous miscarriages or abortions before my conception?
- Had you lost any children before me? Was I a surviving twin?
- What was the nature of yours and my father's relationship at that time?
- How were you feeling physically, emotionally, and spiritually?

Pregnancy

- How was your pregnancy? Were there any complications or health concerns?
- What kind of support or lack of support was around you at the time?
- What kind of medical care did you receive?

- How did you feel physically, emotionally, and spiritually?
- How was your relationship with my father during this time?
- How did other family members feel about my coming?

Birth:

- What do you remember about my birth? (natural, induced, surgery, etc.)
- Were there any complications?
- Were you anaesthetized, induced, were forceps or a vacuum extractor used?
- Were there cord complications?
- How did you feel about the birth?

Write in your journal what you learn about your birth and how you feel about what you have discovered. Share with your partner. If you find that disturbing or overwhelming emotions are triggered as you gather any of this information, you might consider talking about this with a healing professional. You may need to process and heal some of the physical, psychological, and spiritual wounding that could have occurred. According to those who are working in perinatal and paranatal psychology, 85% to 95% of the population experience some degree of prenatal and birth trauma. If you resonate with this notion, seek out a professional who specializes in healing birth trauma. (see *Resources*)

Healing the Mother Wound

As we begin to consider becoming a mother or father, it is important to explore our relationship with our parents. Contemplating parenthood naturally triggers our own childhood memories, and may even activate recall of our own conception and birth. For this reason, the mother/child relationship, beginning at conception (if not before), is significantly important to understand and, if needed, to heal. However, this ritual can easily be adapted to healing your relationship with your father or any individual who had an important impact on you and your life.

This exercise is not about making anyone wrong, but rather provides an opportunity for insight and understanding and ways to heal the mother/child dynamic with our own mothers before we set out to be parents ourselves. Deep healing work with our parents (whether they are alive or deceased) allows us to disengage from multigenerational mythology and to break self-destructive, negative, and unhealthy patterns. Often both our mother's wound and our own is very similar. Becoming more aware of the wounds that may have transpired in the womb, at birth—or at any time for that matter—is the beginning of creating new patterns.

In your *sacred space,* sit comfortably. Allow whatever you are sitting on to fully support your body. Now focus on your breath as you breathe in and breathe out. With your eyes closed, ask yourself, "Where do I hold my mother in my body?" Just notice. Be aware of any sensations arising in your body. Notice any discomfort or agitation. Bring your focus there. Keep breathing and noticing. Ask again, "Where do I hold my mother in my body?" (If you don't connect to any bodily sensations, pay attention to your thoughts or any visual images). The idea is to not push or force any of this, but to allow your experience to be whatever it is. Now ask, "Where do I hold my mother wound?" (I usually get a tickle in my throat—my wound is related to holding back my voice.)

Once you connect with a bodily sensation or sensations, thought or image, etc., ask it aloud or silently, "What are you trying to communicate to me?" Or ask, "What is it that you are trying to show me?" Listen for the response. Try not to force a response. And if nothing comes right away, just practice *deep breathing* for a few moments. Remember that with any of these exercises there is not a perfect way or one single way to do them. Be patient and and trust that the answers will come in the most perfect way and at the most perfect time.

You can also ask, "What is it that I need to know or do to heal this wound?" (What often comes to me whenever I feel that particular tickle is, "It is safe for me to have my own voice. It is safe for me to speak my truth.") Or you might get an insight about working through a specific issue with your mother. Your responses may be different each time, or you may find the wound site and dialogue the same. Have faith and trust in your own inner wisdom and know that it is guiding you in this healing process. For deeper exploration and healing see *The Mother Wound Healing Ritual*.

In addition to connecting with a potential wound, you also may discover where your mother or father express themselves through you in a positive way (sometimes I can see my mother's artistic talents in my hands or feel my father's love for writing through my own).

STORIES

In the gathering of these stories I was reminded of how important our stories are. Whether we are gleaning wisdom from the beliefs and customs of indigenous cultures, or captivated by stories told to us by our family and friends, it is our stories that link us deeply to one another. No stories do that better than the ones that sing the songs of our babies and children.

Traditional
- Our desires, wishes, and dreams can call forth a child. In fact, some individuals believe that there are souls crowding around us who are begging to come in, and that they are just waiting, often impatiently, to be invited.

- Many traditional cultures believe that the soul of the child visits her future mother and/or father in their dreams—often guiding and instructing them in preparation for conception.
- The Hopi of the American Southwest travel to a specific side of a sacred mountain, where prayers are offered for either a baby girl or baby boy.
- It was believed by the indigenous tribes of the Northwest that the Northern Lights were unborn children playing and laughing in the spirit world.
- From where do babies come? Legends, folk tales, mythology, and art render explanations beyond the physiological. Whether carried in the mouth of a stork or cradled in the arms of *Night And Her Train of Stars* (a painting by Edward Robert Hughes depicting a mother/angel figure who is carrying and surrounded by a sky full of little cherubic beings), the arrival of our babies is pure magic dancing in the spheres.

Personal

In spiritual circles there is an expression and belief that children are "closer to the light," meaning that children are intimately connected to the spirit world, heaven, God, the Divine. After all, it is the place from which they have just come. Nothing can confirm this more than when a child spontaneously draws or talks about the "other world"—especially in reference to the arrival of a future sibling. The following true stories illustrate the poignancy of children's instinctive knowing and wisdom.

- In a drawing, a three-year-old child colors a baby in the belly of his mother several months before the conception of his baby sister.
- A three-and-a-half-year-old child announces to her parents that she is going to have a baby sister. She knows

this because her unborn sister has been "playing" with her for "days and days and days"!

- One little boy said that his "new brother" (a brother who was yet to be conceived) told him what he wanted his name to be when he was born.

Meditation, creative visualization, and dreams can also offer powerful information and experiences.

- During a vision quest in the Rocky Mountains, my friend Ken was told that he would be the father of a baby boy sometime soon. His wife, Marilynn, received a similar message around the same time, over a thousand miles away. Ken and Marilynn conceived their son several months later.
- Another friend, who had been trying to conceive a child with his wife, kept seeing a beautiful, black-haired little girl who appeared to be his daughter, in a series of dreams. My friend and his wife, both fair-haired and blue-eyed, were puzzled by the physical characteristics of this little girl. But a year and a half later, after several unexpected events, my friend and his wife adopted an orphaned baby girl from India.
- Within the first few weeks of dating, Colleen and Jeff knew that they would marry. And when they began talking about having a child together, they received what they felt were "visitations" from the natural world, which offered its blessings. These "blessings" included a little bird perching next to them and listening when they first talked about their desire to have a baby together; Colleen having a dream of a beautiful bear four days before going on their first camping trip together; and then seeing a beautiful bear twice on that camping trip together! Colleen and Jeff conceived their baby daughter the following month.

- Personal healing work was something that Elizabeth had never been moved to do. That is, until she endured three miscarriages. A friend had recommended that she work with a psychotherapist who specialized in grief. In their work together, Elizabeth uncovered layers of unresolved grief and loss linking to her past history. Elizabeth is certain that the deep healing work that she committed to doing ultimately helped to "clear the way for a baby" in her life. Elizabeth and her husband are now happily chasing very active twin boys.

RITUALS, CEREMONIES, AND CELEBRATIONS

Rituals, Ceremonies, and Celebrations provide ways to deepen and imprint growth and healing, while celebrating and honoring our lives. Their primary purpose is to awaken our awareness of how interconnected we are to all of life. To help us reconnect with our soul's song, while honoring and welcoming the song of our child.

Our lives are composed of rituals. Throughout history, mankind has used rituals as a way to connect with the forces of nature and the universe. Tiziana De Rovere, in *Sacred Fire,* defines ritual as "a sacred ceremony performed with a specific intention . . . such intention is expressed through a sequence of meaningful actions, often symbolic—to open pathways between our conscious, deep psyche, and the Divine."

Rituals may be simple, elaborate, founded in tradition, personally designed, planned in advance, or inspired in the spirit-of-the-moment. They may be performed alone or with a community of family and friends.

I was fascinated to learn that the word ritual comes from the Latin word *ritus* or river. "Our life force or spirit is like a river that flows through every living thing. When we take time to mark a passage, we are dipping into the river of life." *(Danc-*

ing Up The Moon, by Robin Heerens Lysne). As we "dip into the river of life," we touch into the depths of our being, while the depth of our being touches us.

In the context of carrying a baby into the world, I think that rituals provide a structure, or *sacred ground,* for helping us feel more present and grounded amidst all of the dramatic changes that we are experiencing. And rituals help to bring a deeper quality of awareness to our everyday life, instilling the ability to recognize the extraordinary in the ordinary, the sacred in the mundane.

All in all, the *Rituals* and *Ceremonies* (I use these words interchangeably) are meant to help facilitate and integrate our healing work at the deepest levels, while enhancing our awareness and appreciation of our life. It is from this place that we can more clearly hear the echo of our child's song, as well as our own.

Celebrations (which may be included as part of our rituals) have less structure. They offer a way to help us honor and express appreciation for our sorrows and joys, while strengthening our relationship to ourself, to our loved ones, and to life as a whole.

As you come to any *Ritual, Ceremony,* or *Celebration,* read through it first. Notice if it moves you. Do you connect with it? Can you imagine yourself doing the ritual? What are you drawn to? What doesn't feel comfortable or true? How can you personalize it? Pay close attention to your responses, as the way that you respond will inform you whether or not this particular ritual is appropriate for you. Also, give special attention to the ones that you might adamantly resist, as they just may be the ones that will facilitate the deepest learning.

Ultimately, *Rituals, Ceremonies, and Celebrations* are meant to inspire and encourage you to create your own experiences for healing and celebrating your life. Always trust your intuition and inner wisdom when it comes to selecting, designing, and performing them.

Blessing the Sacred Space

You will need: candle, matches, smudge stick or incense, a small bowl of rice, and a small bowl of water.

Once you have created your sacred space, it is always lovely to bless it. A house blessing or a sacred space blessing is meant to purify the space physically and psychically. The cleansed space can be filled with loving prayers and chants that offer protection and guidance. Although fresh new energy can always be brought and created here, this space can serve as a powerful holy place amidst the chaos of our life. And because you will be exploring the depths of your being there, it is essential that you feel safe and secure. A client of mine described her sacred space as "sitting on the lap of the Divine."

When you are ready to do the blessing, select a time when you will not be interrupted or rushed. Sit comfortably. Take three nice long and full breaths. Allow the breath to center and calm you. Light a candle. And then express to yourself silently or out loud, the intention of this ritual, e.g., I have come here to purify and bless this sacred space. Any energy, negative or otherwise, that does not serve my higher good or support my spiritual growth, is not wanted here.

Many Native American cultures burn sage or sweet grass for purifying and cleansing. Herbs, incense, and candles can serve a similar purpose. At this point, move to each corner of your sacred space, carrying the sage or incense, and silently or aloud say: May this space be a safe place where I can be myself honestly and genuinely. Where I can be with the vastness of my thoughts and feelings, especially those from which I wish to turn away. May this be a safe space where I can meet the disowned parts of myself; where I can work toward healing my soul wound, and where I can discover my soul gifts. May it be a place where I can feel loving and where I can feel loved.

Then sprinkle droplets of water and/or toss some rice around the space (each grain of rice symbolizes a prayer). Listen to music that moves you, read words by someone who inspires you, or drum, chant, or sing your soul's song. Bless your sacred space as it blesses you.

Note: This blessing ritual can be adapted and used for *Creating a Sacred Space, Couple's Shared Sanctuary,* and *Creating a Family Altar.*

Weeding the Garden Ritual

This ritual expands upon the *Weeding the Garden* exercise. Adapt the exercise into a ritual for releasing anything! Be clear in stating the intention of this ritual. Write a letter to whatever you wish to let go of (guilt and shame, a hurtful relationship, an unhealthy life-style, unresolved grief) and discard it in the recommended ways (see *Weeding the Garden* exercise). Invite loved ones to participate and/or witness your healing. Once you have discarded that which you wish to release, find a symbol (a picture, sculpture, a newly planted pot) that represents your new state of being. Place the symbol where you can see it every day as an affirmation for new growth.

A Couple's Healing Ritual
(Using The Mandorla)

Before doing this ritual, you will need to do the *Mandorla Exercise* or include the exercise as part of the *Couple's Healing Ritual.*

In your couple's sanctuary, or anywhere else where you feel safe and comfortable, create a mandorla on the floor or ground with rocks, stones, pinecones, seashells—anything of the earth. Outline the shape of the mandorla, creating the two overlapping circles, making it large enough so that you and your partner can sit inside it. One of you will be Partner A in the right-hand circle; the other, Partner B, will sit in the left-hand circle. Take turns giving voice to that particular quality of your part of the mandorla, as determined in the mandorla exercise. Take a few moments to speak about who you are and why you are here in this part of the circle, first Partner A (e.g., I am loyalty. I feel very strong and committed to my family and to my growth, etc.), then Partner B (e.g., I am resentment and anger. I hold all of our unresolved angers). Dialogue back and forth to each other now. At some point, talk about the fear or any other feelings that you might have about being synthesized together. For example, Partner B might say, I'm afraid that if we merge together, you will become lax again, and I'll just have to keep containing all of the years of resentment and anger, and Partner A might say, I just want to talk about the joys of having a baby . . . I don't want to deal with you and the other scary stuff.

When you feel ready, both Partner A and B leave their respective places in the circle and sit together in the almond-shaped section of the mandorla. Now look into each other's eyes, hold hands, and talk about what you can create together. You might note that being in one extreme or the other is not particularly helpful, and talk about how in joining together you create something even more powerful (e.g., that our unwavering loyalty and passion about growing together will help us better know, more truthfully, our feelings about becoming parents). If you already did the *mandorla exercise,* bring a symbol that represents this healing statement to the ritual; if not, take a few minutes now to talk about what symbol you might create together (e.g., draw and paint a mandorla, make a drum, a poem, or a talking stick that can be placed in the *couple's sanctuary* or on the *family altar).* Conclude the ritual with a prayer of blessing.

The Mother Wound Healing Ritual

You will need: a symbol representing the mother wound, a symbol representing a loving mother (The Divine Mother, the goddesses, Mother Earth, someone you admire), sage, a candle, matches, a small pitcher of water, a bowl, a hand towel, and a piece of fabric to wrap and discard the mother wound symbol in. You can either do *The Mother Wound Exercise* prior to doing this ritual, or include it as part of this ritual (the exercise helps you connect with your mother wound).

In your *sacred place,* lay out before you the symbol(s) of the Mother Wound and the symbol of the Loving Mother. You can burn the sage for cleansing and purifying your *sacred space.* As you sit, center yourself with your breath. Light the candle and then state your intention for the ritual as a prayer. "I willingly release this wound and its destructive and hurtful effect on my life. I let go of my grief, anger, etc." Say whatever you need to say about this wounding. Then pick up the mother wound symbol and blow into it three times, while imagining that you are expelling the damaging and injurious experience and beliefs into the symbol. Wrap the symbol in the fabric and place it to the side. You can either discard it now, as part of the ritual, or do it later. Now slowly pour the clean water from the pitcher into the bowl. Set the pitcher down. Dip the fingertips of your right hand into the bowl. Gently dab the beads of water on the crown of your head, your forehead, eyes, ears, and mouth. Think of the water as holy water purifying and clearing away that which you have perceived and experienced as destructive and hurtful to your soul's evolvement. Dip your fingers again and touch that place on your body where you have held or internalized the mother wound. Say something like, "With this water I cleanse and heal this wound."

Now take the Loving Mother symbol and hold it in your hands. Bless this image and what it represents to you. You might talk about the gifts that your own mother has given you. Bring the symbol to your heart. Breathe in the healing imagery. Imagine your heart softening and expanding. Allow all of your senses to experience whatever you are feeling. Express gratitude for this healing.

Calling Forth the Child

Inspired by the African tribeswomen who sit and listen for the song of their future child, this ritual offers a way to "call out" to your unborn child and invite her into your life.

You will need: smudge stick or incense, candle, drum, materials for writing a letter, painting, or drawing a picture. If you choose to make a collage, have your materials gathered in a basket (e.g., scissors, glue, photographs, magazine pictures, scraps of fabric, heavyweight paper).

You may find that it is more meaningful to do this ritual alone, or you may choose to invite your partner and your other children. Your sacred space, shared couple's sanctuary, the family altar, or a special place outdoors are ideal settings for this ceremony. Purify this space with a smudge stick, sage, or incense. Light a candle. Open the ritual by stating the purpose, that you have come to this sacred place to invite a child into your life. You can read from anything that expresses the sacredness of this ritual. You might select a reading from *Motherprayer*, a lovely book that offers traditional poems, prayers, and meditations for the pregnant woman, by Tikva Frymer-Kensky. The following excerpt is from "In The Waters Of Intercourse—A Babylonian Birth Incantation."

> . . . The way is open for you,
> the way is clear.
> She will assist you,
> She the creator,
> She who created us all.
>
> To the locks she will say,
> "Be loosened,"
> The door sills are apart,
> The door is raised.

As a desired child,
Bring yourself forth.

You, along with your partner and children, can also compose a letter, create a collage, paint or draw a picture to the unborn child, inviting him or her into your family. Simply drumming, chanting and/or meditating can be powerful. Creating an experience of your intention with a sense of sacredness sends forth a loving conscious message to souls who wish to manifest in bodily form.

Place your letter, artwork, etc. on the family altar, or some other place that is highly visible to you. Each time you connect with the image(s), say the prayer spoken in this ritual, sing your chant, or meditate on a symbol—remember the sacred invitation.

2

Listening Under a Tree
CONCEPTION

The Zuni of the American Southwest have a traditional practice in which a singer greets and honors the rising sun with a song.

The Zuni's song to the sun is much like our "calling forth" to our unborn child. As the Zuni singer listens for the sun's response, and as the African woman, who was introduced in this book's *Introduction,* sits beneath a tree in the bush listening for her child, we, too, need to listen for our future son's or daughter's soul song.

This quality of *listening* during this time is characterized by a shift in our awareness, which we might call "conception consciousness." Our senses become heightened, and we experience a natural inclination to look more truthfully at our life. This form of conscious *listening* can dramatically pop open a pathway to a wellspring of inner resources. And although these resources are always available to us, we suddenly begin to discover ways to better access them. We begin to tap into the wisdom and knowledge that resides within, and to the wisdom and knowledge that surrounds us in every moment. Cultivating this way of *listening* gives us the capacity not only to hear our child's song, but to hear our own as well. It is where we can greet and be greeted by one another in our most intimate and genuine way.

There are a myriad of techniques to help us develop our *listening* skills, and I have suggested some of those ways in the exercise section. However, the most important thing to note is that *listening* is not just one more thing that you must conquest and conquer. *Listening* is allowing ourselves to rest and receive—to nourish ourselves in the stillness, while surrendering to nonaction.

Merely contemplating having a child begins a rite of passage that is unequivocally the most profound of any you will navigate through all of the days of your life. Whether the conception is unexpected or planned, or whether we conceive biologically or through adoption—embodied in every seed and egg is the mystery of life.

Murshida Vera Justin Corda, an educator, counselor, and sufi teacher, speaks of this mystery in her lovely book, *Cradle of Heaven*.

"Just as the image of the full-blown rose cannot be imagined in the tight green bud; as the miracle of the baby at birth cannot be imagined to grow from the microscopic union of sperm and egg; conception remains a sacred and beautiful mystery.

The mystery of conception awes and subtly leads to higher spiritual attunement between man and woman, while stimulating the search for deeper understanding of the purpose of life. This same act of divine creation within humankind has been occurring for eons, yet to each couple who fully experiences the miracle of union, it is like again becoming the first parents in the garden of Eden."

The fantasy of a new life with a child brims full of great promise and excitement. But if we allow ourselves to venture closer to all of our feelings, we discover the fear and ambivalence as well. To pay attention and *listen* to what is rustling within leads us to that "higher spiritual attunement" and the "search for a deeper understanding of the purpose of life."

Whether you are first-time parents (biologically or adopting) or preparing for a second or a third child, each pregnancy and birth is as unique and extraordinary as the soul of the child who is forthcoming. That soul, combined with our own soul's purpose and the larger forces at play, sets into motion physical, mental, emotional, and spiritual changes that transform our lives forever. At this spectacular time, *listening* becomes a precious resource.

Just as the dawn's golden rays gently awaken a sleeping world, *listening* stirs us up out of a trancelike sleep, where we have taken safe refuge. The trance, a survival mechanism devised long ago, has become one of the ways to cope in a world that is unable to welcome our true essence. The pain endured from this lack of honoring is often the source of much of life's suffering. Our soul cries out from the heart of the wound within, but our soul's song is overcome by a deep hypnotic sleep.

As potential parents we can either continue to drift in the trance, or wake up. Of course, waking up is not the easiest choice. We will be called to look at our life with unwavering honesty and truthfulness. We will be forced to journey through the unchartered waters of our psyche. Yet, it is an extraordinary opportunity to know ourselves better. Although this may sound self-serving, our commitment to our personal growth takes great courage and bravery. As we heal, our mind, body, and heart soften and open more fully to the astonishing experience of welcoming and loving our children.

The *calling forth* in Chapter One asks us first to contemplate and envision the creation of our garden. Once we have done this we loosen and uproot the weeds and stones in the garden's soil. Now we can properly and lovingly plant the seeds.

When we take the vows of conscious parenting, we begin, even before physical conception, the creation of the growing environment (physical and spiritual) for our child. What kind of setting will that be? With strong *listening* skills we access the wisdom and guidance of our inner voice, the voice of the divine, and even the voice of our unborn child. Seeding the garden then becomes a co-creation of singing souls.

Perhaps you are already intuitively practicing the skill of

listening. Perhaps it was *listening* to your inner voice or maybe even the soul of your child that led you to this book or a healing modality that supports your spiritual growth and development at this pivotal time.

Some people believe that due to the grave nature of our current global affairs—political and religious war, violence, disease, famine, and environmental concerns—strong, willful, and focused souls are choosing to be born; spiritual warriors coming to heal the soul wound of our planet. Who knows, maybe they have already begun their healing work on this physical plane, as they urge us, their future parents and caretakers, to look at our lives with compassionate truth and to reconnect with our own lost souls.

CULTIVATING SKILLS

Listening enriches and builds upon the practice of *being present*—both of which facilitate being more awake in our lives. *Healing our Grief* and practicing *Forgiveness* facilitate deep healing work and ultimately foster a more vibrant and loving environment in which to invite and welcome our future children.

Listening

I could easily write an entire book on *listening.* For Westerners on the "go, go, go," the practice of being still, let alone *listening,* can feel unnatural and awkward. In fact, it may feel so uncomfortable that our first impulse will be to "go" even faster. However, the practice of being still can offer gifts beyond our wildest dreams.

When I worked as a counselor and lecturer at a holistic health spa, I regularly gave a talk on the benefits and rewards of carving out quiet-time in our life. The topic was inspired by the hundreds of people I worked with who suffered from a plethora of complaints: migraines, anxiety attacks, sleep and eating disorders, high blood pressure, lack of energy, depression, and other miscellaneous aches and pains. Aside from their physical discomforts, many described their life as too busy and too stressful.

After discussing the value of stillness, physically and mentally, I would gently guide the participants in a five-minute relaxation exercise. Everyone was invited to sit quietly, breathe, and listen to the sounds around them, beginning with their breath. For most, the exercise was extremely relaxing. Yet when it came time to figure out how they might begin such a practice in their daily life, many were at a total loss. Many claimed not to have time. Some even confessed that the prospect of being "still" for too long was, at best, disturbing.

This reaction isn't surprising, really, given the action-packed movement of our lives. We have evolved into a culture besieged by overwhelming and consuming stimuli that meet us at every turn and from every direction. Yet our insatiable thirst for that magic "something" outside of ourselves perpetuates the chase. We crave what we know or what seems to comfort us, however short-lived or unsatisfying. And like any addictive illness, the chase, the getting, and the fix are merely a desperate attempt to fill the cavernous psychological and spiritual holes—to soothe the soul wound.

Of course what we are truly longing for is that part of ourselves from which we became disconnected so long ago. It is in the stillness, I believe, where we can connect with that lost part of ourselves and begin to remember the melody of our most genuine self, our essence—our soul's song.

And yet, though we strain
against the deadening grip
Of daily necessity,
I sense there is this mystery:

> *All life is being lived.*
> *Who is living it, then?*
> *Is it the things themselves,*
> *Or something waiting inside them,*
> *Like an unplayed melody in a flute?*
> —RAINER MARIA RILKE

Rilke's poetry speaks to the deep pain, "the deadening grip," that we all, on some level or another, suffer from. Somewhere inside, we feel our soul crying out "the unplayed melody." It is in the quiet, in the stillness, in the silence that we just might hear the thunder of our soul's presence.

Listening shares with *mindfulness* and *being present* the practice of giving our full attention to the moment. As we hone the skills of *listening,* we enhance our capacity to be more mindful and present, and as we practice *mindfulness* and *being present,* we strengthen our ability to listen more effectively. Be it *listening* to the voice of a partner, our child, our inner voice, or the voice of the spheres, our lives can be profoundly enriched and deepened by merely *listening.*

The seventeenth-century German priest and poet Angelus Silesius speaks so beautifully of this extraordinary quality of *listening.*

> God is a pure no thing
> concealed in now and here
> The less you reach for him
> the more he will appear

HEALING OUR GRIEF

For those of us who have experienced loss through miscarriage, stillbirth, abortion, or the death of an infant or a child, the sorrow and pain is unimaginable. Other losses related to childbearing—infertility, giving up a child for adoption, losing a child in a custody suit, unsuccessful adoptions, traumatic birth, birthing a physically disabled or ill baby—can be equally heartbreaking. And although it may seem strange or inappropriate to present grief work in a book about birth, this couldn't be further from the truth. The distance that we create from any of our feelings—especially grief—is the distance that we will create in our relationships to ourselves, to our partner, and to our child.

I specifically am highlighting grief because in a culture that idealizes and romanticizes youth and beauty, dealing with death is either rushed, glossed over, or not responded to at all. We are not supported or taught how to deal with death, or any kind of loss, for that matter. Consequently, our body, mind, and heart become the containers of a lifetime of lost dreams, anger, hurt, and pain.

The loss of a child, infant, or fetus can be one of the most devastating and most difficult to heal—no matter how that loss is incurred. The guilt, blame, shame, and remorse that we feel is only intensified by the lack of support and sensitivity of our world. And for many women who have endured any form of abuse—whether it be sexual, physical, verbal, or emotional, self-inflicted or inflicted by another—the pain of not being loved and honored in a respectful way often becomes buried deep within the womb. The womb, meant for bringing forth new life at its fullest potential, becomes a cold and forbidding desert, numbed by a lifetime of unexpressed feelings. In my work around fertility, I have found that difficulties in conceiving or bringing a baby to full term can often be linked to this unresolved pain.

Yes, grieving is absolutely essential for cleansing and healing our wounds from any kind of loss. And for those of us wishing to conceive, carry, and give birth to a baby (physically and spiritually) the work that we do around grief may be one of the most life-altering and life-giving experiences of all.

Forgiveness

Forgiveness is a stepping-stone along our healing path that can be extraordinarily liberating. *For it gives to you* freedom from past hurts and pains held tightly within. Forgiveness does not, in any way, mean condoning hurtful actions inflicted by others. But holding of any kind (rage, resentment, bitterness) can severely restrict the potential for new life. You may need to first examine the uninvestigated and unexpressed feelings that lie beneath that which we wish to forgive. Anger, sadness, grief, and other emotions must be acknowledged and honored before moving on to the next step. Forgiveness is a process of healing and may embody the gamut of feelings before any sense of resolution comes. This is a process that can not be forced or manipulated. Be gentle and patient with yourself.

The exercises provided in this chapter can begin to help free yourself from what blocks and hardens our own hearts. Through this process of doing our healing work we naturally expand our ability and capacity to understand, appreciate, and love ourself and the souls who are coming into our world as our children.

EXERCISES

The following exercises offer some of the ways in which the skill of *listening* can be cultivated and applied. Merely practicing the *Guided Meditation on Listening* will sharpen and expand your capacity to *listen* with all of your senses— from *listening* with your ears, eyes, nose, skin. . . .and even with your toes! *Listening to Your Inner Voice* shows you how to specifically apply your *listening* skills as an interactive healing tool.

Unveiling Our Fears, Grief Work, and Jack Kornfield's *Forgiveness Meditation* deepen our individual work and will help us better welcome and honor our children for who they are, rather than project our unresolved issues onto them.

Writing a Letter to Our Unborn Child, Nondominant Handwriting, and *Creating a Family Altar* offer wonderful ways to begin to bond with your child and experience your new role as parent.

A GUIDED MEDITATION ON LISTENING

In your sacred space or anywhere that you would like to practice listening, sit comfortably with your spine erect. Close your eyes. Focus on your breath. Allow your breath to breathe in its own natural way. Breathing in. Breathing out. Just sitting, resting, and breathing. There isn't anything that you need to know or do in this moment. There isn't any other place to be right now. Just here. Breathing, sitting, and resting. Notice the surface which you are sitting and resting on. Feel it holding you and supporting you. Feel free to adjust your body. Breathing in and breathing out. So natural and effortless. Easy breath in. Easy breath out. Notice any sensations that arise. Merely noticing. Focusing again on the breath. Breathing in and breathing out. Notice the sound of your breathing. Breathing in and breathing out. Merely noticing. Needing to do nothing but to allow the breath to do what it knows to do. Resting, breathing, and noticing. Listening to the sounds around you. Noticing the sounds just beyond your body. Listening with all of your senses. Always merely noticing. Allowing the sounds to move through you. Breathing easily. Now allow a minute or two for sitting quietly. When ready, gently return to the breath. Allow the breath to slowly bring you back into your body. Easily coming back into the present moment. Take a nice deep inhale through your nose. Exhale slowly and evenly out through your mouth. Slowly open your eyes.

LISTENING TO YOUR INNER VOICE

Allow yourself to sit comfortably. Close your eyes and focus on your breath. Let your mind and body relax. Breathing in and breathing out in your own natural rhythm. There is no need to force or push, merely to allow. Allowing the breath to do what it knows to do. . . .so easily, so effortlessly. Each breath relaxing you even more. Breathing in. Breathing out. Allowing yourself to be where you are, just as you are. Noticing any sensations that arise. Breathing through the sensations. Noticing any thoughts that arise. Breathing through the thoughts. Allowing yourself to always come back to the breath. When you feel ready, ask your inner wisdom for guidance around any question that you might have. (If you wish, you can phrase your question in this way, "What is it that I need to know about this particular issue?") Once you have asked the question, it is essential that you *listen* for the response. The message may come to you in words, an image or symbol, an animal, or you may experience, through your senses, a feeling. *Listen* and be patient, as you can't rush wisdom—in fact, the response may come to you later. If the message coming seems unclear, don't be shy to ask for clarification. Allow for at least five minutes. During that time repeat the question, listen, and breathe.

When you feel as though enough time has passed, express gratitude to your inner wisdom. Gently bring your awareness back to the breath. Each breath carries you back fully into your body and into the present moment. Whenever you are ready, slowly open your eyes.

Take a moment following this meditation to write down

your experience, as the process of writing can offer further illumination. Please do not be disappointed if "nothing" seemed to happen. Our questions alone begin to move us to a deeper place along our healing path. And don't be surprised if the guidance that we are looking for appears in the most unlikely place and at the most unlikely time. Stephen, a friend of mine from New York, says that he often finds the response to his inner questions in the words found in ads on the sides of buses that zip up and down the streets of Manhattan. Many times, when I turn on the radio, I hear lyrics that provide an insight to some issue that I am having questions about.

So after asking a question, always pay close attention to your world around you. You never know how your inner wisdom or the voice of the Divine—or whoever else you believe is guiding you—will appear!

Unveiling Our Fears

Our life as an individual is changed forever the moment that we begin to think of bringing a child into the world. Change, even "good" change, brings forth fear in capital letters! The following exercise is designed both to acknowledge and to investigate the fear that naturally arises during this time, so it can be an ally (bringing forth invaluable inner feelings that may be otherwise inaccessible) rather than merely a source of pain and discomfort.

In your sacred space create your own ceremony or meditation for investigating the following questions. You can write your responses in your journal or record them on an audio cassette or even videotape them. These questions can first be individually answered and then shared and/or answered together as a couple. Express all of your fears, no matter how silly and irrational that you might think they are.

• What are my fears about having a child?

- What are my fears about becoming a mother or father?
- What are the fears that I have about my partner becoming a mother or father?
- What are the fears that I have about my relationship, especially in the context of becoming parents together?
- Do I have any fears about how having a child might affect my relationship to my family and to my friends?
- Do I have any fears about how having a child might affect my career, or my freedom and independence?

You might want to do this exercise over the course of several days. And as your fears are revealed to you, talk about them with your partner, a friend, or a healing professional. Write your fears down in your journal or in a letter. Draw, paint, dance, or make music to express them. The important thing is to acknowledge their presence. As the wonderful spiritual teacher Ram Dass might suggest—invite your fears in for tea. Have a chat. Learn from their company. Embrace what they have come to teach you. See *Unveiling Our Fears Ritual* for deeper work.

Grief Work Exercise

This exercise is for the purpose of getting in touch with our unresolved grief. If you are unsure of what your grief looks like, or whether or not you are carrying any at all, you might find this exercise extremely useful.

Cut a long piece of paper from a roll of art paper found in an office or art supply store. Draw an outline of your body. Or have your partner or an older child trace the outline of your body for you onto the paper. Have a box of crayons or colored pens nearby. Read the following guided meditation and then do the exercise, or record the meditation on an audio cassette, play it back, and do the exercise with your own voice. After you have drawn the outline of your body, sit comfortably and close your eyes. Focus on your breath. Breathing in. Breathing out. Easy, relaxing breath. There is no other place to be than right here. Breathing in. Breathing out. Breathing easily and effortlessly. Feel the breath moving and flowing through your chest. Heart opening and softening. Breathing into yourself. . . .breathing out, breathing into this moment, breathing into this healing time for you. Now imagine in your mind's eye the word LOSS. Notice what arises in your mind. Breathing through whatever comes. Just breathing and noticing. Noticing the sensations in your body. Breathing through those sensations. Knowing that whatever comes or doesn't come is perfect. Notice if anything is happening anywhere in your body. Just notice. Then ask yourself—where do I hold loss or grief in my body?

Open your eyes and write, draw, or color in the area where you are holding the emotion that you are working on. Always trust your first response, even if it doesn't seem to make sense to your rational mind. While you are doing the exercise, continue to notice what is coming up. Write or color that in as well. Close your eyes once again. Take a few nice deep breaths. Bring your attention back to your heart. Breathing in and breathing out. Now ask, "What is it that I need to know or do, to help me heal this pain?" Open your eyes and jot down your response. It may be one word, or you may simply experience a feeling (e.g., I need to rest, create firmer boundaries, say no more often, give myself permission to self-nurture). Write or draw your response on your outline. Give some thought to how you might integrate what you have learned into your life. For example, if you need to nurture yourself more, what and how might you establish that in your life? Write down your thoughts and a possible plan in your journal.

If nothing seems to come to you in this exercise, either wait and listen, or be open to receive that message in some other way and at some other time. You might even try connecting with your loss and grief by adapting some of the other exercises offered in the book *(Nondominant Handwriting, Dialoguing, Listening to Your Inner Wisdom* exercises). There are many ways to grieve. You may grieve over a long period of time, or you may symbolically release the grief in a specially designed ritual (see the *Index Of Exercises And Rituals).*

As in all of the exercises offered in this book, you might consider following up or enhancing your work with journal-writing, bodywork, hypnotherapy, one-on-one counseling, art therapy, movement—any modality that you personally connect to. Always allow your intuition and your heart to guide you. This is an excellent exercise for exploring other feelings as well, such as anger and fear.

Writing a Letter to Your Unborn Child

One of the ways to connect to your unborn child is to write him a letter. In your sacred space or outdoors during the new moon (the time for new beginnings) put on some favorite music, light a candle, and compose a letter to your future child. The letter can be written, drawn and/or painted in your journal. Ask any question that will help you honor and welcome your child.

First, ask yourself the following:

- What are your dreams, hopes, and fantasies about becoming a mother or father?
- What are your dreams, hopes, and fantasies for your child?
- What do you hope to offer this child as his parents?
- What do you imagine this child will teach you?

Now ask the child:

- Is there anything that I (we) need to know to prepare for you?

- Why have you selected us to be your parents?
- What is your soul's purpose?
- How can I (we) help you fulfill this purpose?
- Is there anything else I (we) need to know to honor your coming?

If for any reason you find yourself having difficulty with any of these questions, consider doing the *Listening to Your Inner Voice* exercise, *Communing with The Soul of Your Child Meditation* or the *Nondominant Handwriting Exercise* below.

Nondominant Handwriting Exercise

Using nondominant handwriting exercises is a surprisingly powerful healing tool. I have used variations of this technique in both my personal and my psychotherapy practice for years, and for a wide variety of purposes. In my work with individuals living with life-challenging illnesses, I have found writing to one's disease and having it respond through the nondominant hand can be exquisitely insightful and helpful. In the context of conception, this exercise may be useful in knowing how to better prepare for an incoming spirit, especially if you are having difficulties becoming and/or staying pregnant.

Nondominant handwriting works because it bypasses the analytical right brain—which, although an indispensable asset, is in fact limiting. Accessing the left hemisphere of the brain through this technique opens a doorway into the vast and boundless resources within, be it the wisdom of our higher consciousness, the divine, or perhaps the wisdom of the unborn child.

I have a journal full of letters that I have written using this technique to explore physical discomforts, relationship conflicts, and unresolved childhood issues. The technique proved to be most helpful during my difficulties getting pregnant and staying pregnant; I know that I was guided somehow by my son, long before he was conceived.

Whether the responses coming through the pen and your nondominant hand are from your inner wisdom, the wisdom of the heavenly spheres, or the wisdom of an unmanifested being, is not really important, as far as I am concerned. What is vitally important is that we have expanded and opened ourselves up to a voice that is longing to be listened to.

Sit in your sacred space or anywhere that you feel comfortable and safe. Select a person, a challenge, or any issue that is troubling you. In your dominant hand write a letter addressed to that particular person or issue. Express your thoughts, feelings, and questions openly and honestly. Your last sentence might say something like: "Please let me know in words, what you have come to teach me or show me." When you feel complete, take a few deep breaths, place the pen or pencil in your nondominant hand, and respond to the first letter. You may feel clumsy and even silly writing with your nondominant hand, but stay with it. Write the first thing that comes, even if it doesn't seem to make sense. When people get stuck, I tell them to just write about that: "I'm stuck, can not find a word, this is so silly. . . ." You may find that you will need to try this exercise several times before you feel more comfortable. Or you may surprise yourself when you find that after writing, "I'm stuck—why is she asking me to do this????" something begins to happen. You can write letters back and forth until you feel that you have received a helpful message. And by the way, although this technique offers a venue for doing the deepest of work, it does not always have to be a solemn experience. Our inner life secretly yearns for a pen pal!

A Forgiveness Meditation

This Forgiveness Meditation can be found in *Buddha's Little Instruction Book,* by Jack Kornfield. It is a beautiful meditation on opening up our heart and releasing the pain of the past. As indicated earlier in this chapter, you can not force, rush, or manipulate forgiveness. Forgiving is a process, which opens and unfolds over time. This meditation can be useful as a practice towards healing wounds of our past, while freeing ourselves of that which can ultimately paralyze and hinder our growth.

To practice the following forgiveness meditation, let yourself sit comfortably, allowing your eyes to close and your breath to be natural and easy. Let your body and mind relax. Breathing gently into the area of your heart, let yourself feel all the barriers you have erected and the emotions that you have carried because you have not forgiven—not forgiven yourself, not forgiven others. Let yourself feel the pain of keeping your heart closed. Then, breathing softly, read aloud or record the following words from Jack Kornfield's meditation. Allow the images and feelings that come up to grow deeper as you repeat them.

FORGIVENESS OF OTHERS: Silently or aloud, say "There are many ways that I have hurt and harmed others, have betrayed or abandoned them, caused them suffering, knowingly or unknowingly, out of my pain, fear, anger, and confusion." Let yourself remember and visualize the ways you have hurt others. See and feel the pain you have caused out of your own fear and confusion. Feel your own sorrow and regret. Sense that finally you can release this burden and ask for forgiveness. Picture each memory that still burdens your heart. And then to each person in your mind repeat: "I ask for your forgiveness, I ask for your forgiveness."

FORGIVENESS FOR YOURSELF: Silently or aloud, say "There are many ways that I have hurt and harmed myself. I have betrayed or abandoned myself many times through thought, word, or deed, knowingly and unknowingly." Feel your own precious body and life. Let yourself see the ways you have hurt or harmed yourself. Picture them, remember them. Feel the sorrow you have carried from this and sense that you can release these burdens. Extend forgiveness for each of them, one by one. Repeat to yourself: "For the ways I have hurt myself through action or inaction, out of fear, pain, and confusion, I now extend a full and heartfelt forgiveness. I forgive myself, I forgive myself."

FORGIVENESS FOR THOSE WHO HAVE HURT OR HARMED YOU: Silently or aloud, say "There are many ways I have been harmed by others, abused or abandoned, knowingly or unknowingly, in thought, word, or deed." Let yourself picture and remember these many ways. Feel the sorrow you have carried from this past, and sense that you can release this burden of pain by extending forgiveness when your heart is ready. Now say to yourself: "I now remember the many ways others have hurt or harmed me, wounded me, out of fear, pain, confusion, and anger. I have carried this pain in my heart too long. To the extent that I am ready, I offer them forgiveness. To those who have caused me harm, I offer my forgiveness, I forgive you."

Let yourself gently repeat these three directions for forgiveness until you feel a release in your heart. For some great pains you may not feel a release, but only the burden and the anguish of the anger you have held. Touch this softly. Be forgiving of yourself for not being ready to let go and move on. Forgiveness cannot be forced; it cannot be artificial. Simply continue the practice and let the words and images work gradually in their own way. In time you can make the forgiveness meditation a regular part of your life, letting go of the past and opening your heart to each new moment with a wise, loving kindness.

Creating the Family Altar

A place in your home or yard might be designated as the family altar—an idea introduced in *Celebrating the Great Mother,* by Cait Johnson and Maura Shaw. It's a special place (fireplace mantel, windowsill, a piece of furniture) where family members bring something of themselves—artwork, photographs, poems, stones, a tree branch, or flowers. It's here that you can gather together to pray, sing, drink tea, chat, or hold a family meeting.

If you have other children you could come to the family altar to ask them what they think about inviting a baby brother or sister into the family. Of course, you have to be prepared for the truth! When contemplating having a second child, a friend of mine asked his four-year-old son what he thought about having a baby sister or brother. After a brief pause and a long sigh, the child looked into his father's eyes and said, "I'd rather play golf."

The family altar can also be a place where, individually and/ or collectively, the spirit of a child is invited to the family. You could do this by saying a prayer, writing, visualizing, or meditating on the child. A gift could be placed here at this time or later.

Note: You can easily adapt this exercise into a ritual *(Blessing the Family Altar Ritual)*. Have the family members bring their meaningful object(s) to the ceremony. Bless the altar with a prayer, chant, song, or a poem that you have selected previously, or compose something new, spontaneously in the moment. You might have each family member talk about what purpose they hope this space/family altar might serve. If one of the purposes is to welcome a new family member, place on the altar some type of symbol (a sculpture, picture, drawing of a baby or child, or a small bowl with rose petals) of the family's invitation to the unborn spirit. This is a wonderful opportunity and a way for children to participate in inviting the new soul into the family. My son writes letters to the angels, asking for his sister (whom he has already named) to come and join us. We all eagerly await her coming.

Sacred Ground

Sacred Ground is a variation or an extension of your *sacred space* and the *family altar*. I think of it as *sacred space* on wheels. It is simply keeping a connection with your sacred space and/or family altar no matter where you are. You can do this in a tangible way by carrying a sacred object with you that is used in any of your rituals, such as a polished stone, crystal, or medicine bag, or by merely connecting to the spirit or energy of this special place, through imagery and through your senses. I have a faded red Native American wool blanket that I sit on when I meditate in my sacred space. It is the same blanket that I might use in a ritual, or throw over my chair while sitting and writing these pages (at my writing desk or in front of the computer). I have known some women who have brought their *sacred ground* (sacred objects from their altar, a blanket, gifts given to them and their baby in a ritual) to the hospital when they gave birth. For them, the *sacred ground* provided a womblike feeling during the process of labor and birth. In fact, the *sacred ground,* imbued with loving, supportive, and healing energy, seemed to be helpful to all those attending the birth, including the birth partners and other children, when present. One expectant father was told by several hospital staff members that they wanted to stay in the room where his wife was in labor, because it felt so "wonderfully healing and amazing" there.

FERTILITY

Not being able to conceive and/or bring a baby to full term can be physically, mentally, and emotionally painful. Because this situation can feel so distressing, isolating, and sometimes even hopeless, it seemed important to include the following information that could be supportive and helpful.

The statistics say that one out of six married couples of child-bearing age has trouble conceiving and completing a successful pregnancy. Some experts hold poor nutrition and stress as largely responsible. Others blame various medical conditions, which can only be treated with drugs and surgery.

If you are experiencing any issues involving infertility, I strongly urge you to explore (along with all of your other options) the mind/body/spirit connection in relationship to becoming pregnant and birthing a baby.

Niravi B. Payne, founder of the Whole Person Fertility Program and author of *The Language of Fertility—A Revolutionary Mind-Body Program for Conscious Conception,* has counseled hundreds of clients from all over the world who have experienced fertility issues. Payne, a psychotherapist, biofeedback specialist, and pioneer in mind/body fertility therapy, believes that reproductive problems, including miscarriages, difficulty in conceiving, and low sperm count, can be directly linked to attitudes, beliefs, and family dynamics that reach back into our childhood. Using meditations, visualizations, and journal-writing, Payne has helped her clients break through the emotional barriers to conception. She dispels many of the myths ("old eggs," "unexplained infertility") while offering practical methods to help individuals become more conscious in reclaiming their health and wellness. Payne also believes that labeling anyone as infertile is extremely hurtful and can interfere with having a successful pregnancy and birth.

Many of the exercises and rituals in *Welcoming The Soul of a Child* can help heal issues that may be hindering your natural fertility. For example, unexpressed grief regarding any loss, especially a miscarriage or an abortion, can impede our natural ability to conceive and give birth. *The Grief Work Exercise* and *Healing Waters* or *Planting a Tree in Honor of Loss* rituals offer invaluable steps toward healing the pain of that loss.

Acknowledging how our wellness is affected by the interconnectedness of mind, body, and spirit can greatly open up the possibility for healing many of our health issues, including infertility. (See the *Index for Exercises and Rituals* for other healing processes.)

The following is one of many wonderful visualizations offered in Payne's book, *The Language of Fertility.*

NATURE'S ODE TO CONCEPTION

This visualization is specifically designed to celebrate your fertility and to help prepare your endometrium (the mucous membrane lining the uterus) to receive a fertilized egg and hold the pregnancy to term.

You can either have your partner or a friend read the following to you, or you can read it aloud into a tape recorder, accompanied by reflective music that you find soothing and comforting.

Begin by making yourself comfortable, shifting your weight so you can feel fully supported, whether you are sitting or lying down.

Let your eyes gently close. Note if your head, neck, and spine are in alignment. Take a cleansing breath; inhale as fully as you can, pause, and then breathe out. Take another deep breath and as you exhale, imagine you are sending it down into your belly. Take another deep breath and as you exhale, send the warm energy of your breath to any part of your body that feels sore, tense, or tight. As you continue breathing deeply, release any tension with each exhalation. Feel your body slowly ease and relax, loosening and letting go of all tense areas. Allow yourself to feel safe and comfortable, relaxed and easy.

Now picture yourself in a beautiful forest. The forest is the abundant fertility of the primordial Earth Mother. It is rich with dark green foliage. Overhead there is a brilliant, warm sun. Take a deep breath. The blue sky is crystal clear. As you walk through this lush, highly vegetated green forest, there is an underlying green moss carpet spread on the rich soil. This forest is so fertile with life, so abundant with life. Listen to the excitement of the birds singing, calling to one another in the sweetest symphony in the world. It is nature's symphony, an ode to life, an ode to creation, an ode to fertility. In your mind's eye, see an absolutely exquisite sun. Visualize the sun's rays streaming forth through the foliage of the trees, entering your heart and warming every space within your being. See the rays then streaming out of your heart's center and back into the world. Listen to the birds singing a song of fertility, of life, renewal of life; just listen for a few moments. Breathe deeply.

You can hear a brook somewhere in the distance, flowing over the rocks and twigs, adding its sounds to the most exquisite symphony of sound and movement. Now . . . see beautiful flowers. Look at their colors as you breathe in their fragrances, sending the essence down into your womb, opening, receiving, and giving forth. The sun is continuing to send its healing rays throughout every cell, tissue, and muscle of your body, bringing its rays right into your womb.

As you feel the warmth of the sun's rays penetrating deeply into your uterus, see the rays streaming forth from your womb out into the world, healing the world. There is a beautiful circular energy pulsating throughout—into your body, then out, into your body and out. Every part of your body feels so relaxed. As with all of nature, your body is ready to receive and give forth, receive and give forth.

In the midst of this wonderful process of receiving and letting go, realize that anytime there are feelings of sadness, anger, tension, worry, anxiety, they, too, are part of nature. Nature is not only sun; it is also wind, rain, and storms. Nature is hurricanes, tornadoes, floods, and blizzards. All of this is nature. Add some protection from the storms of life for the new life you want to grow within you. See yourself placing your future baby in a beautiful pink bubble. This isn't just any pink bubble: it's an exquisite crystalline bubble that is full of life-enhancing oxygen to protect the baby in the moments when you experience emotional reactions to difficult situations. You can say to the baby, "I'm here to protect you. I can't promise that I will be the world's best mom. I will make mistakes. I will not have cleansed everything negative from my psyche, but I welcome your arrival and I am committed to doing my very best." When you feel you are ready, slowly open your eyes.

After this visualization, write down in your journal your own message to your future baby with a prayer that the spirit and the body unite to form the creation of the baby you have long waited for.

STORIES

When collecting the traditional stories for this book, I came across Jacqueline Vincent Priya's book, *Birth Traditions and Modern Pregnancy Care*. It's a fascinating book exploring women's knowledge and beliefs about conception, pregnancy, labor, and birth in traditional cultures around the world. Priya, a mother of three, sociologist, author, and researcher, founded and runs The Birth Traditions Survival Bank from her home in Malawi. And although Priya does not suggest that we adopt or copy the customs practiced in any of these cultures, per se, she does hope that we can preserve them through writing them down and appreciating the wealth of wisdom that they do offer.

"Giving birth was, for [women from traditional societies], an experience in which no distinction was made between the physical, psychological, social, or spiritual: where each aspect was viewed as equally necessary and equally valid. The physical acts of conception, pregnancy, and birth were but one aspect of a cycle in which social, individual, and divine forces all played a part. This cycle mirrored the cycle of birth, growth, and death which they saw in the natural world around them and derived from their traditional wisdom about the nature of life and death. For these women to give birth was to participate in the mystery of life on earth, and this was recognized not only by themselves, but by the people who helped them give birth, as well as the rest of the people in the community in which they lived."

Traditional

My intention in sharing the following stories (some from Priya's book and others found in other research) is to capture the spirit of how many traditional societies view conception far beyond the egg being fertilized by the sperm.

- The Dinka tribe in Sudan believe that conception is the outcome of the work of God, the ancestors, and man. It is believed that the child belongs to the deities, the ancestors, and those still to be born. The ancestors seem to possess the strongest influence as it is they who can ensure the continuation of the family tree.

- The Karen (one of the hill tribes in northern Thailand) believe that the child's spirit determines the nature of its life and its death long before birth.

- Also in Thailand, conception is not considered successful unless the soul of the unborn child is lodged inside the womb of the mother during intercourse. At the time of conception, the pregnant woman may have a dream which may reveal the gender of the unborn child, as well as what kind of person she or he will be when grown up.

- On Trobriand, a small group of islands in the Pacific, it is believed that spirits to be born drift around in the sea after coming from the spirit world. These spirits are invisible, although they may be seen in a trance or heard by a fisherman. An ancestor spirit takes the spirit child to the mother and weaves it through her hair. On the tide of the mother's blood, the child is carried into the woman's womb.

- The Aborigines of Australia believed until recently that the spirits of their children came through food eaten. At conception the presence of the spirit was often discovered in a dream by the mother and/or father. Later, the food in which the spirit child was carried becomes the child's conception totem and a very significant part of the child's spiritual life.

- At conception in the Middle East, the Angel of the Night carries the soul around to view its future life and then returns it to the mother's womb, where it will remain for the duration of pregnancy. When the child is born she/he forgets the world from which she/he has come.

- The image of a stork delivering a baby to its rightful home originated in northern Europe. Apparently, the legend grew from how storks tenderly care for their young, sick, and aged, combined with another ancient tradition which held that the souls of unborn children dwelt in watery places—as do storks.

- In Latin America the moon goddess, Yemaya, also the patroness of motherhood, was usually asked to be helpful with fertility. In one such ceremony a pomegranate is cut in half and covered with honey. The name of the individual wishing to conceive is then written on a piece of paper and placed in between the halves. Yemaya is asked to help this person to be as fruitful and as healthy as the pomegranate. A blue candle burns every day for a month, starting with the first day of the menstrual cycle.

Personal

- A friend of mine, who had a history of miscarriages and who "ached for a child," found herself stirred from a deep sleep for several consecutive nights by what sounded like a "haunting melody sung by a mature female voice." The moment my friend was fully awake however, the singing abruptly stopped. In meditation she was told that the song was a healing chant and was being sung by her unborn daughter. My friend conceived shortly after this and gave birth to a gorgeous little baby girl nine months later. The melody, which she hummed during labor and birth is her daughter's favorite "song."

- A three-year-old boy proudly announces that he is going to have a baby sister. His mother is certain that she is not pregnant, but a pregnancy test later confirms the little boy's matter-of-fact knowing.

- A five-year-old boy was fascinated for months with baby tortoises and drew a series of pictures of them hatching from their eggs. This was at the same time that his parents were, unbeknownst to him, trying to conceive a second child. One day he drew a baby tortoise totally emerged from its shell—joining a family, including mother, father and an "older boy tortoise." Nine months later, the little boy (now a bit older), mother, and father joyfully greeted a new baby sister.

- Several years before she conceived her first child, a woman felt compelled to buy an antique rocking chair. She says the chair became her sacred place where she did meditations for healing a childhood wound, which "cleared the way for my son to be conceived and born."

RITUALS, CEREMONIES, AND CELEBRATIONS

Healing Waters, Planting A Tree In Honor Of Loss, and *Planting Seeds* are poignant ways to move toward healing wounds from loss. This meaningful work is integral to creating the open and loving welcome that our children so richly deserve.

A Lovemaking Prayer and *Listening for the Child's Song* acknowledges and honors their coming.

Grieving Loss

The following rituals offer an intimate and sacred way to grieve and mourn any loss. They may be particularly useful for healing a loss concerning childbearing.

HEALING WATERS

You will need: uninterrupted private time, a bathtub, candles, vinegar, the essence of lavender or lavender oil, and any related thoughts pertaining to this particular loss, from a favorite poem, song, or book, or words or chants of your own. This ritual is particularly healing following bodywork, or any other inner work which evokes deep emotions.

Dim the lights and make a bath with approximately one tablespoon of vinegar, which is a good detoxifier. Get into the bath and relax for a few minutes. As you light a candle, say out loud a prayer that states the purpose of this ritual, such as: "In this sacred water and in the sacred moment, I invite (whomever you wish from the spiritual realm—it may be especially healing to invite the spirit or the soul of the child that you lost) to assist me in letting go of and healing this grief wound. I willingly and lovingly release the pain. May the warm healing waters of the Universal Divine cleanse and purify my body, mind, heart, and soul."

Now read the words you have selected, chant or sing. It is extremely important to give yourself complete permission to mourn in any way that you feel moved. Surrender to your emotions. Scream, wail, howl if you feel the impulse.

When doing this ritual for mourning my miscarriages, I intuitively began to chant the following for each loss:

Baby, baby
I'm so sad
You're the one I never held
Freedom now
Freedom now
Out to heaven's warm embrace
Carrying you to your perfect place
Eternally loving your soul with grace.

When ready, drain the tub and imagine the grief being released. Once the water is gone, refill the tub and add several drops of lavender oil. (Lavender is wonderfully soothing and calming.) Now relax quietly in the healing water. If you wish, play peaceful music or create a new chant or prayer in celebration. Marcia, my dear friend and "soul sister" who has experienced her own loss around childbirth, wrote me this beautiful poem, which I then read out loud in the soothing and healing water.

This loss may be thought of as
a visitation
from a wise old soul
stopping by for a moment
to rest and renew
in your welcoming body . . .
then moving on.
Shared lessons, cleansing tears, and
clarity of vision
remain forever—
beyond the tears—
and leave a deepening beyond words,
a greater connection
than any attachment on this
earthly plane.
I'm sad with you
and grieve beside you . . .

our little angels or spirit guides, those souls
join the others
and we stay here, together,
for now.

Close the ritual by saying a blessing of gratitude. Drain the water and slip into something very cozy. Write or draw about this experience in your journal now or later. Rest.

PLANTING A TREE IN HONOR OF LOSS

Planting a tree in honor of a rite of passage is an ancient practice. It seems only natural, given the tree's wonderful symbolism. The planting ritual can be applied to a myriad of ceremonies. For this reason, you will find variations of this ritual throughout the book. I love trees, so any opportunity to plant one, as far as I'm concerned, benefits us all and Mother Earth tremendously.

This ritual can be one done alone or shared with your loved ones. You might think of it as holding a memorial service. You may be grieving the loss of a fetus, infant, or child, or the promise of giving birth biologically. You may be experiencing the pain resulting from a complicated birth or unsuccessful adoption. Or you may be grieving the changes incurred from separation or divorce, and its impact on the time and way in which you are allowed to be with your child(ren). You may be grieving the loss of your innocence, a dream, or the hope of resolving a conflict with another person who may be unwilling to heal your relationship or who has passed away. There are endless ways that we experience loss. I suggest that you select a loss that seems most relevant to your quest to become a parent (a miscarriage, an abortion, giving up a child for adoption, infertility, death of a child, unresolved issues from childhood). Intuitively you will know where you need to focus your healing.

You will need: a site for planting, a tree (a bush or plant is fine, as well), planting tools, and a symbol of that which you mourn.

Open the ritual by stating your purpose—for example: "Today, I come to this place on my healing path, where I willingly and lovingly honor, release, and free myself of this particular pain and loss." Then take the symbol, and while holding it or placing it in the center of the ceremonial space, imagine that it contains the grief, hurt, or anger that you wish to release.

When you are ready, blow three breaths into the symbol and place it in a piece of cloth or a paper bag. You can discard the object in the trash, bury it (not where you are planting the tree, however) or burn it (now or later). When doing this you can say something like—"By letting go of this object (or pain), I now make room for the possibility of positive new growth in my life. The planting of this tree symbolizes and manifests the rooting and blossoming of that which will come forth." If you want a child, mention that as part of the ritual. "In letting go of the grief, I now make a healthy, nourishing and loving environment in my body and in my life for my future child. I invite this child into my (our) life now."

Plant the tree, in a place that has already been prepared. Once firmly in the ground, water it well. Think of the soil, the oxygen, the sun, and the water as ideal growing nutrients for what you wish to grow. Express gratitude to those elements— earth, air, fire, and water. Express gratitude to yourself for having the willingness to do this ritual. And then give thanks to whomever and to whatever you feel assists you on your healing path.

Planting Seeds

Planting seeds in a garden or in a clay pot is a wonderful ritual that symbolizes change and new growth. If the season permits, prepare the ground and plant a tree, the ancient symbol of life (this tree needs to be different than the one that you planted in the ritual *Planting a Tree in Honor of Loss).* If you don't have a place or a way to plant a tree, you might arrange for permission to plant one in a park or on someone else's property. And of course, you can always purchase or adopt a potted plant or tree for indoors.

You can invite your loved ones to this ceremony, or keep it private and small. Have your planting tools and seeds or plants nearby. Gather those participating in a circle around the planting area. If you haven't readied the garden, do so now. (See *Weeding the Garden.*) If you are planting seeds, have those participating collect some of the seeds in their hand. If planting a bush, plant, or tree, have your guests bring a pebble or small stone.

Open the ceremony by talking about the purpose of this ritual. If you wish, read something that you have written or from a meaningful selection of poetry or prose. Then ask each person to silently or verbally say a prayer for new life—imagine breathing that prayer into the seeds for the garden or into the roots of the plant or tree. (You can also imagine breathing the prayer into the small pebbles and stones, which can then be placed loosely atop the soil). Plant the seeds or the tree now. Holding hands around the newly seeded garden or planted bush or tree, allow those participating to share their prayer, thoughts, or how they might volunteer to watch over this newly planted life. End this part of the ceremony by blessing those who have gathered and the life growing within the earth.

Sharing food and music together is always a lovely way to culminate any sacred ceremony. And by all means, if you have children, include them in this ritual. They love to plant seeds and watch them grow. It is also a wonderful way for them to express a little bit of their own soul in the welcoming process.

A Lovemaking Prayer

Parents-to-be are holy gardeners. Coming together to create a child is one of the most magnificent graces that can ever be bestowed upon us. This ritual is meant to honor that gift, as well as to consciously invite a child into our life.

Please feel free to modify and personalize this ritual. The idea is to create a meaningful experience for you, your partner, and your future child. And if you have already conceived (unplanned or not), you and your partner can still honor the conception of your child by performing this ritual as if you were in the process of conceiving. The growing fetus and the soul of your child always benefit from your heartfelt intentions.

Think of creating a sacred space, sacred altar, or sacred ground prior to the ceremony. Select a comfortable and intimate place—your bed, cushions on the floor, or a secluded and private place in nature. Decorate this space with flowers, silk scarves, and candles. Create a center in this ceremonial space by laying out a blanket, velvet fabric, or a scarf. Bring nature objects (try to utilize all four elements—earth, fire, water, and air), a smudge stick or incense, lavender or rose water mist, and a gift for the child. You can also bring a bowl of water with floating candles, a basket of rose petals, and a marriage bundle, which contains a gift for your partner.

When you and your partner are ready, enter the space together. Light your smudge stick or incense and purify the space. Sit down in the heart of the ceremonial space facing each other. Take one or two nice deep breaths together. Express the purpose of this ceremony. Looking into each other's eyes, share what you appreciate about your partner. Now express what gifts you believe each of you will offer your future child. How do you imagine yourself together as parents? If you feel self-conscious or nervous about these questions or the ritual itself, talk about that as well.

Spray the lavender or rose water mist into the air. Lightly

toss the rose petals upon the place where you will caress and make love. Read a favorite passage from a book, recite poetry, sing, dance, or play music together. Exchange gifts. Then gently dab your fingertips into the bowl of water. Place the droplets of water on your partner's hair, forehead, eyes, mouth, and belly. Say a prayer or blessing to the incoming spirit. Welcome the soul into your lives. Make your gift offering to your child.

Co-create a ceremony that is alive and vibrant in the moment. On that note, always allow for the unexpected! During this ceremony, some friends' lovemaking was abruptly ended when an overzealous smudge stick set off a smoke alarm which summoned the attention of concerned neighbors. While another couple was making love, one of the partners got an excruciating leg cramp, which could only be relieved by applying an icepack. Of course, it is these kinds of incidents that bring levity into the experience, which is sometimes the perfect medicine. Don't hesitate to integrate lightness and play into your rituals, because something tells me that incoming baby spirits want to have fun from the very beginning!

Listening For the Child's Song

This ritual is inspired by various African tribes who have a tradition of listening for the song of their child. In their eyes, conception occurs at the moment when the song is heard.

I imagine this ritual, in particular, as one that can be used throughout the entire life cycle of being a parent—from before conception through pregnancy and birth. In fact, I believe that the essence of this ritual can be an invaluable way to connect to your child throughout his life! Whether you hear the child's so-called song or not, merely sitting and listening is an exquisite way to honor your child's soul.

As we know, there are a multitude of benefits to sitting quietly, the very least of which is it gives us a golden opportunity to restore and renew ourselves, physiologically and emotionally. However, I also believe that sitting quietly and *listening* provides us the luxury of reconnecting spiritually to ourselves, to our life, as well as to our child.

Find a tree to sit beneath, whether outdoors or indoors. If a tree isn't handy, then create a symbolic one with streamers, a sculpture, or a picture. Or you might bring a fallen tree branch, tree blossoms, or leaves to your altar. (If you haven't designed an altar, this is a wonderful occasion to do so. See *Creating a Sacred Space* or *Creating the Family Altar*). Place a gift to the baby's spirit on the altar.

You may perform this ritual once or, if you are trying to conceive, you may choose to do it during each ovulation cycle or during the new moon (the time for new beginnings). The more that you practice the essence of this ritual, the better you will be able to listen anywhere.

You will need: A tree, sage or incense, and candles.

Begin the ritual by purifying the space with the sage or incense. Light a candle. Sit comfortably with your spine erect. Focus on your breathing. Breathe in a sense of ease and quiet. Breathe out any tension or discomfort in the body. Breathe in. . . .breathe out. Once relaxed, say aloud or to yourself the purpose of this ritual, something like, "Here I sit beneath this tree and it is here where I listen for you, sweet child. I welcome your special song. I welcome you." Sit quietly.

Anytime you find your mind distracted, or if you are feeling sleepy, gently return to your breath. Take a nice deep breath in and release it slowly. Do this several times. Restate the purpose of the ritual once again. You can also just simply focus on the word SONG or the words CHILD'S SOUL SONG. Bringing your attention to a word or words can become a chant or mantra. Or think of it as a focusing technique, which helps ground the intent of the ritual. Give yourself uninterrupted quiet and private time to do this ritual. You can always begin with five- to ten-minute sessions, and then work your way up to longer times. Write, paint, draw, or sing about your experience.

If it feels as though nothing has happened, remember *listening* is about receiving. The important thing is to create opportunities for hearing your child's song. Receiving the song is something that can not be rushed. And who knows, maybe the incoming spirit has fashioned a symphony of songs and is merely pondering which one will aptly express this life's story. Or, in an extraordinary choir of voices, he may simply be anticipating his solo part, composed intricately just for him. Or maybe he is just waiting for his backup singers to arrive!

> *Inside everyone*
> *Is a great shout of joy*
> *Waiting to be born.*
>
> —DAVID WHYTE

3

Singing the Child's Song
PRENATAL

Joy to the world,
All the boys and girls
Joy to the fishes in the deep blue sea
Joy to you and me!

Jeremiah was a bullfrog
He was a good friend of mine . . .

HOYT AXTON

We enjoy all different kinds of music at our house. When I was pregnant with my son, I gravitated particularly to the Scottish singer and composer Enya. My husband, on the other hand (who really is a rock n' roller at heart), would massage my moonlike belly, and in his own inimitable style, croon "Joy To The World" to our unborn child. This would always make me giggle, and I'm certain that I felt the little guy inside of me (who at this time we had nicknamed Spike) leap for joy a couple of times.

Do you know that our ears are the first organs to form completely? In Don Campbell's fascinating book, *The Mozart Effect,* he writes, "Today embryologists agree that the ear is the first organ to develop in embryo, becomes functional after only eighteen weeks, and that it listens actively from twenty-four weeks on." Now researchers are confirming how responsive fetuses are to sound. In fact, a fetus will move toward pleasing sounds and recoil when sounds are too loud, chaotic, or harsh.

Campbell, who has researched and studied the effects of music on healing, reveals in his book how exposure to sound, music, and other forms of vibration, beginning in utero, can have a lifelong effect on health, learning, and behavior. Apparently, one of the fastest growing fields of music therapy and intervention involves pregnancy, delivery, and infancy. Campbell tells of various studies demonstrating that women have fewer complications and spend less time in hospitals when incorporating music into their birth experience. A technique called toning, which is similar to humming, can help women dramatically reduce both anxiety and the physical discomforts during pregnancy and birth, and even once the baby has come home.

Talking tenderly, reading a favorite children's story out loud, singing chants and lullabies, and listening to harmonious sounds and music are wonderful and important ways to nurture and nourish your babies before they pop out on their birth date.

The brilliant French physician Dr. Alfred Tomatis, who is an expert on the physiology of hearing and the first in the medical community to recognize that the fetus hears in the womb, writes in his book, *The Conscious Ear,* "The universe of sound in which the embryo is submerged is remarkably rich in sound qualities of every kind. . . . the embryo draws a feeling of security from this permanent dialogue which guarantees it will have a harmonious blossoming."

There is no doubt that sound, vibration, and music dramatically affect the developing baby in utero and after birth. Infants who are prematurely born, have had open heart surgery, or endured numerous other complications at birth, have recovered remarkably well when music is utilized as a healing tool.

Even siblings can share in the healing effects of music on their newborn brothers or sisters. One of the most riveting stories in *The Mozart Effect* concerns a three-year-old boy whose newborn sister was admitted to a neonatal intensive care unit due to complications that had occurred at birth. At one point, the family had been told by the medical team that the baby's death was imminent. Although small children are not allowed in intensive care units, the parents snuck the little boy, who kept asking to see his baby sister, into his new sibling's room. The boy moved toward the bassinet and began to sere-nade the baby with a song that he had sung to her throughout his mother's pregnancy.

> You are my sunshine, my only sunshine,
> You make me happy when skies are gray.
> You'll never know, dear, how much I love you,
> Please don't take my sunshine away.

The next day, the little boy, his mother, and father took their new family member home. She had responded "miracu-lously" to her brother's familiar voice.

Through extensive research and working with thousands of pupils, Don Campbell has discovered that many children have been known to recognize songs, lullabies, and even classical music that had been played to them in utero.

One of the most well-known stories about how deep an impression music makes on the developing embryo is told in Thomas Verny's provocative book, *The Secret Life of the Unborn Child*. It concerns a Canadian orchestra conductor who found that he could effortlessly play certain pieces of music, sight unseen. When he discussed this with his mother, a professional cellist, she said that they were selections of music that she had rehearsed over and over while she was pregnant with him.

In my life I have come across a number of such stories. Some friends of ours were thrown into despair when their second child was born with a serious respiratory condition.

Both the parents and their doctors attribute the baby's "miraculous" recovery to the mother's daily sessions of gently touching and singing lullabies to the baby.

Leesa, a composer and musician, wrote and sang a chant to her unborn child throughout her pregnancy. But it was Leesa's husband, Michael (a composer and musician as well), who immediately following Leesa's unexpected cesarian, soothed their newborn daughter simply with his speaking voice. Leesa, also a music therapist, found the chant to be extremely helpful in deepening the bond with her baby, especially as she recovered from her surgery. The melody, which Leesa now accompanies with a keyboard, continues to be baby Emma Rae's first song choice.

Music played a remarkable role in my own case, as well. After hours of back labor and then a cesarian, my son was pulled from my body. Even in my heavily medicated state, I clearly recall my ob-gyn saying, "Zach, you are a smart little boy, because you knew if you traveled any further down the birth canal you would have gotten into trouble." Apparently, my cord—"unusually long," per the doctor—was wrapped several times around his neck and chest. I also heard our son crying—no, screaming better describes his state of upset. I remember thinking that our newborn's shrill cries must be reverberating throughout all of Manhattan, if not the entire state. I can't blame him, after what he had just gone through. My husband, who was present and very concerned, reached through all of the green masked arms and bodies and quickly brought Zach to his arms. Intuitively, he began to sing, "Jeremiah was a bullfrog, he was a good friend of mine. . . .Joy to the world. . . ." Zach opened his eyes wide, looked straight into his dad's big brown eyes, and stopped crying immediately!

Who says babies are not awake and aware in the womb? Who says we can't deeply connect with our children prior to their arrival on the physical plane?

Our home, now filled with the enchanting fire spirit of a

six-year-old, is also accented with a rather odd collection of bullfroglike creatures (my favorite one being a rather petite creature with huge feet, wearing a fancy set of gold gossamer angel wings). And Zach still leaps for joy when listening to "Joy To The World"—his dad's version, of course!

In addition to responding to sound during the earliest stages of development in the womb, our babies are extremely sensitive to touch. Studies have reflected fetuses moving toward pleasant and gentle touch when their mothers are being tenderly massaged, and moving away from anything that may be intrusive (like an amniocentesis needle). Gently massaging the mother's body has numerous physiological benefits for both mother and unborn child, while at the same time communicating heartfelt love and caring.

Yes, sound, vibration, music, and touch dramatically affect the growing baby. However, what is most important goes beyond the baby's senses being stimulated in a positive way. What enhances these experiences is the quality of love that pours through the music, sound, and touch from parent to child, heart to heart, soul to soul.

So bearing in mind the significance of the emotional, physical, and spiritual well-being of the parents, especially the mother, during pregnancy, it is of paramount importance that we give great thought to how we are welcoming our newborn children. Greeting our babies occurs long before we wrap them in a receiving blanket and hold them in our arms.

There are many excellent books on the physiological and medical aspects of pregnancy (see *Recommended Reading*). In this chapter I want to offer you a mind/body/spirit overview of pregnancy *(Tenderly Tending to the Garden)*, including ways in which you can bond with your baby as well as commune with her soul, while in utero. To prepare specifically for the labor and birth, I have included exercises for selecting your health care professional and for designing a birth plan. There are visualizations for pregnancy and labor, suggestions for self-nurturing and strengthening the couple's relationship, and ways to include the birth partner and your other children in preparing for their new child or sibling. The section on *Rituals, Ceremonies, and Celebrations* provides beautiful ways to honor this exquisite time of passage.

TENDERLY TENDING TO THE GARDEN

As we return to the metaphor of caring for The Garden, please be reminded that the mind, body, heart, and soul aren't really separate entities. Although for the purpose of discussion, I will focus on them one at a time, as always, the goal is to integrate, synthesize, and honor all parts of ourselves.

Body

In addition to tenderly and lovingly caring for your body yourself, it is important to find health care professionals who will honor and respect you physically and emotionally. It is essential that you feel comfortable and trust your prenatal and labor "team." Interview obstetrician/gynecologists, midwives, doulas, and other health care professionals. Please do not be afraid to ask questions. Consider yourself a consumer. I have provided a list of questions or criteria that might be helpful as you make your decisions. There are some questions that do not have right or wrong answers, but rather speak to your own preferences. For example, although I know that there are wonderful male ob-gyns in practice, I wanted a female for my doctor. And I wanted to be assured that the same physician who saw me throughout my pregnancy would be present at the delivery of my son. It was also important to me that my husband would be encouraged to be actively involved during various stages of pregnancy and birth. (During one of my earlier pregnancies that resulted in a miscarriage, my husband was strongly encouraged to wait in the waiting room during my first prenatal examination. The receptionist and nurse were "befuddled" as to why I would want him in the examination room with me!)

Always pay attention to the feelings you get about the support staff of the health care professionals that you are interviewing. Whether you choose a traditional ob-gyn group or a midwife from a midwifery practice, you are basically choosing a family to assist you in one of the most momentous events in your and your child's life. If you don't have the luxury of choosing your health care professional, which is often the case these days with health plans, you can still choose how actively involved you are in your own education, care, and treatment.

At no other time will your body go through such dramatic changes. Prenatal care includes giving meticulous attention to your ever-changing body so that you can best care for yourself and your child. For example, if you are feeling fatigued, be certain to get adequate sleep and rest. If you won't permit yourself to slow down—and I urge you to do so—at least learn how to meditate or do deep breathing exercises. Both practices can rejuvenate the body, mind, and soul, especially if done regularly. When you honor the changes—by appreciating and paying attention to them—you will know what you need to do to best care for yourself and your baby. Trust and listen to your body, your baby, and your inner wisdom throughout your pregnancy and birth; they will always guide you well.

Your doctor or midwife should be versed in dietary needs, but if you feel that you need more assistance, talk to a nutritionist. If you have not omitted harmful and toxic substances from your diet, do so now. Studies confirm that cigarette smoking (and even secondhand smoke), caffeine and drugs, including alcohol, are damaging to the growing fetus. If you find it difficult to stop any self-destructive behavior, especially now, please seek professional help. Your child's quality of life, and sometimes her life itself, depends solely on you making the most responsible choices. You can be light and playful during pregnancy (and by all means do!), but please never take this job lightly.

In this chapter, you will also find a section on designing a Birth Plan. This will give you ideal guidelines for choosing how you wish to give birth. Of course, we have to always allow for the unexpected. But in giving thought to and verbally expressing what your wishes are, you will reclaim your own authority over the birth, which in our culture has largely been taken away. Fortunately, this is beginning to change. First, more and more women are dissatisfied with their past birth experiences and unwilling in the future to settle for what they have been offered. Second, pioneering childbirth educators, midwives, doctors, psychologists, and other healing professionals are helping greatly to make necessary changes by acknowledging the life of the unborn child and advocating for the rights of mothers and babies to have gentle and more peaceful birth experiences. I feel blessed that through writing this book I can bring more attention to their important work, as well as do my part in helping to increase awareness and understanding of this subject that I feel so passionate about.

All in all be gentle with yourself and your body during this time. As Thich Nhat Hanh might say, "Lovingly care for yourself as you would bathe the baby Buddha." Bring a sense of tenderness and devotion to caring for yourself and your growing baby. Hum, sing, chant, and dance as you tend to the delicate seeds sprouting forth in the fertile garden.

Mind

Some people feel that they need to know everything that there is to know about pregnancy and birth, and virtually become a walking and talking textbook on the subject. Others have found it more helpful to educate themselves about some of the basics, but leave it at that. They prefer not to have preconceived notions influence the outcome of what will be their unique birth experience. Ultimately, most of us want to be educated, conscientious, and prepared. Take classes, workshops, attend lectures, and read books that you find helpful, talk to your friends who have children or who are pregnant like you, talk to your midwife and/or ob-gyn. Ask tons and tons of questions. But always come back and check in with yourself. Trust your intuitive mind. The wisdom and knowledge found there is boundless. After all, we have been giving birth for millions of years—that has to stand for something! For guidance on how to access your inner wisdom see *Open Heart Meditation, Listening to Your Inner Voice* and *Accessing Your Inner Wisdom*. To connect with your unborn baby see *Writing a Letter to Your Unborn Child, Dialogue with Your Unborn Child,* and *Communing with the Soul.*

Heart

When we are touched by the miracle of life developing inside of us, little is needed to persuade the heart to open. The heart naturally wants to soften and unfold. But having your heart open doesn't mean that you won't feel fear, sadness, grief, and anger. In fact, you probably will feel those feelings all the more. When we allow our heart to feel open, we spontaneously open to all aspects of ourself. This is one of the reasons why this time of our life is so full of self-reflection and is considered by some to be a time of "crisis." Not only does our heart begin to soften, but our entire armor does as well. Letting go or releasing parts of the hardened shell can feel quite frightening. Yet, if we aren't paralyzed or overwhelmed by what is taking place, feeling vulnerable, a little scared and fragile, can be a good thing, because it is in this place that we are given the opportunity to peek behind the mask, to see and feel our true heart's yearning and truth. Cultivating new skills, such as *lis-*

tening and practicing *being present,* can give us more of a capacity to hold the gamut of feelings that are naturally arising.

You may be tempted to attribute your powerful and sometimes disturbing feelings to the biological changes you are undergoing. Yes, there are major shifts occurring physiologically, and the radically fluctuating levels of our hormones do affect us emotionally. But I'm referring to how the expanding body mirrors our expanding awareness and consciousness. As we create more space in our bodies and lives for a baby, we begin to naturally open up to self-reflection. The moment that we invite the soul of a child into our life our journey begins a new path. A path that forces us to take a more truthful look at ourselves and our lives.

So what can be helpful at this time is to care for your body, mind, and heart with heartfelt compassion. Read inspiring words, listen to touching music, draw, paint, go to holy places that you find in your home, in nature, or anywhere in your community. Be with babies, children, and adults who make your heart full. And of course, fullness of heart can be experienced simply by being present and mindful, acknowledging the extraordinary in the ordinary. Allow your heart to brim full of passionate feelings.

Soul

As we lovingly and steadfastly tend our garden, budding life emerges. While rooting themselves in the rich soil, the tiny seedlings push their way up through the earth's surface—knowing exactly what to do, where to go, how to grow. A force of life defining and expressing itself in every moment. Our child's growth and development is nothing less than a miracle.

Their soul magically touching our own soul—nudging us up out of our trancelike slumber—is another miracle. Do we keep sleeping? Or do we awaken to the fully fragrant scents that surround us? Do we turn over and just pull the covers up over our eyes? Or do we allow the sun's ever-abundant warmth and energy to awaken and enliven us?

Allowing this precious time to move us helps penetrate and pierce through the dense and muddy layers of our psyche— offering an opportunity for our own buds to burst forth; a precious gift from the unborn.

Listening has particular meaning at this stage of birthing a child. Whether we are listening for the soul of our child or that of our own soul, we begin to strengthen and enhance our ability to connect—to all of our life. *Listening* offers an opportunity to deepen our connection to the unborn child (see *Baby Bonding* and *Communing with the Soul of the Child*).

This is an excellent time to develop or further develop a regular spiritual practice. I believe that spirituality is intimately personal and sacred. Thus, it is important that you express this in the way that feels most genuine to you. Chogyam Trungpa, a great Zen master says, "Spirituality is about arousing one's spirit." So, as you create a spiritual practice, think about what arouses your spirit, what inspires and moves you. All your responses guide you. Spirituality, for me, is waking up from a trancelike sleep and being more present in my life, experiencing my connection to all of life. My meditation practice, reading inspiring words, walking among trees, and writing and drawing with my son are some of the ways in which my spirit is aroused.

So whether you worship God, the Goddesses, the Universal Divine, Mother Earth, Buddha, Krishna, Jesus, or Jehovah— or if you experience your spirituality when walking on a beach, feeding ducks in the park, brushing your child's hair, reading inspiring text, listening to music, or sitting quietly anywhere— begin a conscious practice of honoring your connection to your spiritual essence.

Devote at least five minutes every day to this practice. Invite your partner and child(ren) to share this experience with you. Breathe deeply, read, pray, meditate, chant, sing, dance, write, or simply sit in the stillness. Express gratitude. (Read *Parenting as a Spiritual Path* and *Creating a Spiritual Practice with your Children* in Chapter Five).

· CULTIVATING SKILLS

More and more research confirms that prenates are aware, have a consciousness, and are dramatically affected by our behavior, feelings, and thoughts. *Baby Bonding* and *Communing with the Soul* acknowledge and honor this belief, while providing ways to meaningfully connect with our child long before their official birth date.

Visualization is an invaluable tool that can be utilized in a variety of ways and can be extremely helpful during pregnancy and childbirth.

Baby Bonding

Bonding or attachment is the exchange of love and trust that develops between a baby and its primary caretakers. Many indigenous cultures believe that the bonding process begins before birth and continues through life, and that bonding also includes the child's relationship/connection to her father, siblings, extended family, and community.

Of late, our culture is beginning to accept this notion, thanks to pioneering and passionate thinkers, such as Dr. Frederick Leboyer *(Birth without Violence),* who advocate birthing our babies in a more gentle and humane way. Leboyer teaches that from the moment of birth humans need to be touched gently. He emphasizes the necessity of making the birthing environment more peaceful and inviting by dimming the lights, keeping the room warm, eliminating loud sounds, and immersing the newborn in water at body temperature immediately following birth, and then gently placing the baby on the mother's stomach. His teaching has virtually revolutionized the way we bring babies into our lives all over the world.

Beginning in utero, we are communicating with our growing baby. Bringing more awareness to that communication is essential to the way in which we do or do not bond right from the very beginning. The quality of bonding with our child dramatically affects the child's growth and development mentally, physically, emotionally, and even spiritually. Joseph Chilton Pearce, a passionate child educator, says bonding is the "connection that facilitates human's spiritual evolution."

Nondominant handwriting and drawing, journal writing, meditation, visualization, reading out loud, massaging the pregnant belly, listening to music, singing, and gently talking to your baby are some of the ways in which you can physically and emotionally strengthen this budding new relationship. (See *Communing with the Soul of the Baby* in the *Index of Exercises and Rituals*).

Communing With the Soul

There are numerous rich and meaningful ways to commune with the soul of your unborn child. Some of the baby-bonding exercises offered in this book present opportunities to do this. *Communing with the Soul* of the baby takes the connecting to a whole other level, as it acknowledges not only the physiological and emotional presence of a baby, but also honors the spiritual and soul self of the unborn child.

Just like the African tribespeople who listen for and sing the unique song of each new baby, I see communing as our way of listening and singing our child's soul song.

Another culture that believes in the importance of honoring the individual soul of a child are the Dagara tribe of West Africa. Sobonfu Somé, a member of that tribe who with her husband, Malidoma, teaches their ancient wisdom throughout the world, shares how their tribe communes with the souls of their children in her book, *The Spirit of Intimacy*. The real beauty of the book is how Somé's own soul seems to emanate through her words as she teaches about the sacred traditions and stories of her people.

In one chapter, called "Born to a Purpose," Somé explains that when two people are married, they make themselves available for a soul to come through them. The Dagara believe that children belong not only to their parents, but to spirit and to the community. They also believe that even before birth the soul knows what gifts it will bring and what its purpose is. During pregnancy, The Hearing Ritual is performed. The elders of the tribe commune with the soul of the unborn (the unborn speaks through his mother's voice), asking questions such as who is this soul, what is its purpose, and how can the villagers and elders assist it on its journey. Based on this information, the elders honor the arriving soul by preparing an appropriate ritual space where the child will be received and welcomed.

During this ritual the soul identifies a stone (which the elders will later seek out), that contains all of the important information about this particular soul and its life.

Following the birth, the child is surrounded by sacred objects chosen by the elders that will serve as reminders of his soul's life work. And during an important initiation at adolescence, the child is led back to the time of his birth so that he will be reminded of what he was born for.

Similar traditions of communing with the soul of an incoming baby are practiced by indigenous cultures as diverse as the Balinese in Indonesia, the Basque in the Pyrenees, the Cherokee of the American Southeast, the Tibetans in the Himalayas, and the Aborigines of Australia.

Pamela Grace, a gifted healer and transpersonal hypnotherapist, helps mothers and fathers communicate with the soul of their child through trance work. It is a stunning way for the child's soul to talk about her life's purpose, as well as share why she and her parents have chosen to be with each other in this life. When a young couple's baby was born with a rare and critical heart defect, they were faced with making a decision to either take their newborn home to die, or have her undergo three high-risk surgeries that would only give her a fifty percent chance of surviving. It was communing with the soul of their unborn child in a session with Pamela that inspired and gave them the courage to have their daughter go through the surgeries. She not only survived the surgeries, but is a vibrant, happy, and healthy little girl and "bringing happiness" (her life's purpose, as conveyed in the session with Pamela) to all those who know her.

Let us continue to be inspired by these sacred customs and create our own exercises, rituals, and celebrations, which invite us to dance together, cheek to cheek, to the sweet melody of our child's distinctive soul's song.

Creative Visualization

Creative visualization is an effective healing tool being used by individuals, healing professionals, and, more and more commonly, by savvy allopathic doctors. It is an invaluable tool that helps you access your inner resources through symbols, images, and feelings.

The term visualization can be misleading. It leads most people to assume that you can only experience it visually. This isn't necessarily so; for some of us, our sensory strengths may be more auditory or kinesthetic in nature. Some healing professionals use the term "felt sense" instead of visualization, to describe this concept more accurately. But to keep things simple, I will use the more familiar term visualization.

The most important thing when using visualization is to pay attention to all of your senses, but particularly the one(s) that become(s) most fully engaged.

Visualization can be used to relieve a variety of symptoms,

including stress, chronic pain, and general anxiety, and can also help strengthen self-esteem and aid in overcoming an illness. Many of my clients have found creative visualization extremely valuable when working with a life-challenging illness or chronically troubling life obstacles. I have taught this healing tool to my clients and workshop participants specifically for all the phases of birthing a child.

I have provided several visualization exercises in this chapter and in Chapter Four that are helpful for preparing for and giving birth to your baby. I have also included a baby-bonding visualization written and used by Carl Jones, the knowledgeable childbirth educator and author of *Visualizations for an Easier Childbirth*, and *Mind over Labor* (See *Recommended Reading*).

Some of the benefits of practicing visualizations during your pregnancy and for childbirth are:

- Greatly reduced anxiety and fear concerning pregnancy and childbirth.
- Increased ability to relax.
- Enhanced connection with your baby.
- Heightened body awareness.
- A stronger mind, body, heart, and soul connection.
- A positive outlook on the birth experience increases the likelihood of a positive outcome.
- Strengthened ability to access your inner wisdom.
- Greater ability to make decisions that are best for you and your baby.
- Less emotional and/or physical pain of labor.
- An easier transition from pregnancy through birth to taking the baby home.
- Increased confidence and faith in your own abilities.
- A way to commune with the baby's soul.

Exercises

Pregnancy is a time of tremendous change and transition, not only physically, but emotionally and spiritually as well. The following exercises offer support and direction for prenatal care, labor, and birth, as well as help you practice accessing your inner wisdom.

Selecting a Healing Professional

Lucia Capacchione, an art therapist and author of nine books, and Sandra Bardsley, a nationally certified childbirth educator and nurse, have written a marvelous book together called *Creating a Joyful Birth Experience.*

They talk about "claiming the territory" when it comes to childbirth, which means not only being well informed, but making proactive choices about the birth of your child. Do your research and then make clear the kind of service you expect to receive. In this respect, choosing your health care should be no different than buying any expensive item or service. After all, "You are dealing with your body and the well-being of your unborn baby . . . Learn to weigh the benefits against the risks."

In *Recommended Reading Resources,* I have listed information, including videos, that can help you feel more informed about this enormously personal and complex aspect of childbirth. The first thing to do is research your options, taking into consideration your philosophy, where you live, your financial resources, health insurance coverage, previous birth experiences, and special health needs or risks.

Capacchione and Bardsley provide detailed guidelines on how to interview a potential health care professional, first by phone and then, if you're satisfied, in an office interview. In each case, have your questions written down ahead of time. In addition to the specific interview questions, Bardsley and

Capacchione suggest that you may want to consider the following:

- Do I feel comfortable with this person and his or her staff?
- Is their birth philosophy compatible with mine?
- Do I agree with their methods of childbirth and early infant care?
- Do their fees fit my budget?
- What services do they offer (lab facilities, ultrasound, bilingual ability)?
- How many health care professionals are in this service, and do they have nurse-midwives on their staff?
- What are the percentage of caesarian-section deliveries, episiotomies, and other types of interventions (vacuum extractor, forceps, internal fetal monitor, internal uterine catheter, routine IV's)?

I would encourage you to add the following, especially if you are considering a more traditional setting:

- How open and flexible are they to my personal needs and requests? For example, would they be open to having other health care professionals be present during the birth (an acupuncturist, massage therapist, a hypnotherapist)?
- If you are interested in having a water birth, can they make arrangements for that?
- Is a midwife and/or doula (a childbirth assistant) permitted to help in the birth process?
- How do they include and support the father/birth partner? Will he be allowed to be present if an epidural is requested or if a cesarian is performed? Will he be allowed to assist in the birth ("catching the baby" or cutting the umbilical cord)?

Creating a Birth Plan

Creating a Birth Plan means writing down what you want and need for you and your baby during labor, delivery, and early postpartum. The first step in preparing one is reflecting on all of the information that you have gathered and deciding what you want and don't want. It is essential that you communicate what you want; otherwise all decisions will be deferred to the medical team on duty at the time. The ultimate goal is to create a safe and joyful experience for you and your baby, so why not spend the necessary time and effort to clarify what that might mean for you?

Talk over the Birth Plan with your partner, support team, and then with your health care professional. Having the Birth Plan signed by your midwife or doctor assures you that the hospital staff will abide by your requests.

In *Creating a Joyful Birth Experience,* the authors provide several writing and drawing exercises that are helpful in getting the clarity that you need for making these important choices.

There are many decisions to make (hospital vs. birthing center, pain medication vs. no medication, desire to have a midwife and/or birth doula present, warm water immersion for the baby at birth, labor and/or birth in a birthing tub, do you want your other children present, etc.). It is easy to feel overwhelmed. But I urge you to reclaim your own authority in this process. Gather the pertinent information—be informed. Also, practice accessing your own intuition and wisdom. After all, as women we have been giving birth for millions of years. Yet, for a number of reasons, we have surrendered our power to a system that isn't always so kind and sensitive to us as pregnant women, nor to our babies. Fortunately, this is beginning to change because more and more women have been dissatisfied with their prenatal care and birthing experiences.

The following is a Birth-Plan Overview provided in *Creating a Joyful Birth Experience*.

BIRTH PLAN

1. Get clear about what you want

   - Notice your internal voice: What are you saying to yourself? What questions are you asking?
   - Define your beliefs and values about any specific aspect of birth that is important to you.
   - Identify your concerns about birth.
   - Identify what makes you happy or excited about the thought of giving birth.
   - Gather information.
   - Share your thoughts with your support person(s).

2. Decide and make a conscious commitment

   - Get clear and focus on your purpose and goals.
   - Use affirmations like "My partner is" or "I am in charge of taking action."
   - Formalize a Birth Plan (write it out).

3. Take action

   - Discuss your Birth Plan with your support team.
   - Condition your responses. Imagine yourself over and over again succeeding in carrying out your plan.
   - Use others who have succeeded as role models.
   - Talk to your doctor or midwife about your Birth Plan. Get their support for your plan and have them sign it.
   - Make an extra copy of your Birth Plan to take with you to the birthplace. Be sure this copy is signed by your care

provider. Once it is signed, your Birth Plan should be considered to be official orders.

4. Make your goal real

- See yourself having the power to give birth the way you want to.
- Believe in your birthing goal. Imagine it over and over again.
- Physically practice what it will take to achieve your goal.
- Reinforce your physical commitment with an immediate reward.
- Have patience, be flexible.
- Be ready for obstacles to your goal. Make alternative action plans.
- Pay attention to what works and what does not work. Be willing to make minor changes until you reach your goal.
- Don't give up (on your support team, yourself, your body, your baby, or your birth process)!

Note: Organize your wishes and goals into the following categories:

- Normal Labor
- Normal Birth
- Early postpartum care for the mother
- Early postpartum care for the newborn
- What to do about unexpected outcomes (such as caesarian, interventions, trauma for the baby)
- Care for your baby (Note: Make your baby's care plan on a separate page, because after the birth it will go into the baby's medical chart.)

For detailed samples of a Birth Plan, see Capacchione and Bardsley's book.

All in all, devoting time to creating a succinct and complete Birth Plan is a wonderful way to reclaim your feminine power. And even if unexpected situations should arise, having surrounded yourself with an attentive and strong support team—those who are familiar with your Birth Plan and you—will only reinforce and strengthen your ability to face whatever challenge comes your way.

Accessing Your Inner Wisdom

Use this meditation any time you feel the need for guidance and clarity regarding this extraordinary life experience. It can also be extremely helpful once your baby is born, when many questions and concerns about taking care of her will no doubt arise.

Before beginning this exercise, reflect on how you would like to use the imagery. Even if you have a specific question, I encourage you always to make room for the unknown. For it is in the unknown where the greatest treasure can be discovered.

Sit comfortably in your *sacred space* or anywhere that you feel safe and secure. Close your eyes. Take two or three nice deep breaths. Breathe in through your nose and exhale slowly and evenly through your mouth. Feel the surface beneath your body completely supporting you. Continue to allow the breath to relax you.

Now imagine yourself in a peaceful place in nature. It can be anywhere. It may be somewhere you have traveled in reality, or perhaps only in your imagination. Allow all of your senses to experience the beauty found here. As you look around, you notice a specific place that feels and looks particularly inviting. You naturally gravitate there, at your own pace and rhythm. As you move closer, you realize that this is your very own sacred sanctuary or sacred temple. You are completely safe and protected here. Allow all of your senses to experience this place. Notice the lighting, the colors and shapes of this environment. Breathe in the fragrances. Listen for the sounds here. Savor the tastes. Feel this place on your body. Feel and see the sanctuary's or temple's qualities of beauty and peace. Somewhere here you find cushions of velvet, a blanket, or the soft earth to sit upon. Where you sit is your power spot. It is here that you feel yourself surrounded by your loved ones, your ancestors, power animals, angels, guides, midwives, and healers—those who come from the earth and those of the spiritual realm. You know that it is in this sacred time and place that all questions can be asked and answered.

Put forth a specific question, or simply ask, "Is there anything that I need to know that can be helpful to me and my baby during this part of our journey together?"

You can also call forth your unborn child. Ask her, if she wishes, to meet you in this sacred place—a place where she can communicate whatever she wishes to. Your child may appear as an infant naked, swaddled in a receiving blanket, or may even appear as an older child. Or she may come to you as a symbol, such as a flower, a color, a bird, or a four-legged animal. You may simply experience a warm lovely feeling, tender and gentle. However she appears, be open to her message. Listen and express thanks.

This visualization will naturally unfold in the way that is most personal and meaningful to you. When you feel complete, take in a nice deep breath through your nose. Exhale slowly and deeply through your mouth. Become aware of your body. Become aware of your breath breathing through you. Allow the breath to carry you back to a more wakeful state. Slowly open your eyes.

Pregnant Body Beautiful

This visualization can be found in Carl Jones's book *Visualizations for an Easier Childbirth*. It offers a way to honor the beauty of your pregnant body and instill confidence in your ability to give birth naturally.

Relax completely, body and mind.

Focus your attention on your breathing, your breath flowing in and out.

Dwell just on your breathing for a minute or two. Follow your breath in and out without trying to control it. Each breath out melts tension away, leaving you more and more relaxed.

Enjoy the feeling of complete relaxation.

Now let your breathing become a little deeper, a little slower, without forcing the breath in.

With each pause, tell yourself that you are entering a deeper, more relaxed state of body and mind.

Now imagine that your in-breath is a soft, radiant, golden light.

Imagine that you are breathing this golden light directly into your womb.

Imagine that the radiant light is filling your womb with health-giving energy.

As you continue to breathe this soft light in, imagine that it begins to radiate outward from your womb to fill your entire being.

Let yourself drift into even deeper relaxation, body and mind, as the radiant light fills your being.

Now imagine that the light is radiating out from you in all directions, a beautiful golden aura or halo.

If you wish, imagine the light is radiating out from you to surround your mate. Let it radiate farther and farther from you until it fills your entire home. Dwell on the image of the soft, radiant light filling your being and expanding in all directions around you for as long as you wish.

Now center your mind in your womb.

The womb is the source of all the changes that are taking place within your body, in your emotions, and even in your home right now.

Imagine that you are able to look within your womb.

Look at your baby: head down in a beautiful shimmering sac filled with crystal-clear fluid, in his or her own private universe.

Look at the beautiful curly bluish white umbilical cord.

Follow the umbilical cord to the placenta attached to your uterine wall.

Imagine the oxygen and nutrients flowing from your body through the placenta, down the umbilical cord to your baby.

Tell yourself: I am able to supply all that my baby needs to grow and be healthy.

Consider what your body has done.

If you can do what you have done already, you can surely labor normally.

Tell yourself: I am able to labor in perfect harmony with nature.

Thank your body for the miracle it is working and will continue to work.

When you are ready, count slowly to five, stretch gently, and open your eyes.

Communing with the Soul of Your Child

Dialogue with the Unborn Child Meditation

The following breathtaking meditation comes from *The Child of your Dreams,* by Laura Huxley and Piero Ferrucci. They introduce the meditation by saying, ". . . whoever you are and whatever your difficulties may be, you are hosting the most wondrous of all developments. Thus, if you can take even five minutes a day to think good thoughts, listen to your favorite music, or nourish yourself in any way you want, your kindness will be multiplied a thousandfold and become an organic part of a person's being for years to come. Five minutes of care is worth years of well-being."

In the imagery that follows, you, the future mother or the future father, will be led to meet your unborn child and dialogue with her. Should you decide to do this imagery together, please remember not to give each other ideas or suggestions. During this meditation, silence is of the essence. It will be a very special dialogue, because the unborn, though human, does not yet belong to your world and knows nothing of your reality. It will be like a dialogue with a being from another planet, living in totally different conditions than your own. And yet this being is infinitely close to you, it is a part of you. For the time being its destiny is your destiny, its body is your own body, therefore a subtle communication can begin to happen. The only way to make this dialogue fruitful is for you to make yourself as receptive as he or she is, and to listen deeply, consciously, openly.

Close your eyes, relax for a few moments, and pay attention to your breathing. Don't force it, but, feeling you have all the time in the world, let it get deeper and slower. As you pay attention to your breath, you become more attentive. For the time being, leave behind your daily cares, your opinions, your habits, even your needs. Let your breathing take care of itself. You are silent consciousness.

As a silent presence, you find that your awareness is becoming more vast, deeper. You are open to what is and receptive in all directions. There is nothing verbal about this awareness. Naked awareness, stripped of all concepts, is particularly sensitive to even the subtlest feelings, sensations, and intimations.

As pure consciousness you can be anywhere: in the depths of the ocean or on top of a mountain peak, on a deserted beach or in a forest, inside a leaf or on a rainbow, in the center of the earth or on a star.

Of all the possible places within your reach, you choose the dark, enchanted dwelling of the unborn, where you will meet the child of your dreams. You will journey to the mysterious abode where human life begins.

You travel now through layers of flesh and placenta, through the wondrous geometry of cells, through pulsating blood, in veins and dark spaces, through the living factory of inner organs, through amazing landscapes, towards that deep place where life is created.

You reach the place where the unborn is living. A tiny heart is beating; a form is slowly undulating in this liquid medium, suspended in space. The eyes do not yet see the forms we are so familiar with: they are still open to infinity. You have an impression of something powerful and sublime at work here; with precise pace, with timeless knowing, all is developing. You are there, you are conscious. You sense the presence of a being. It is your child.

Take some time now to establish a contact with this presence. You are totally attentive now, open to any message that may come to you.

You listen. The presence of the unborn is itself a communication. You sense its mood, its state of being. As you set your assumptions aside, messages reach you with surprising clarity.

Now the unborn is communicating with you in a more active way.

Listen! It tells you where it comes from.

Listen! It tells you about its life now.

Listen! It tells you its wishes, its needs.

Listen! It tells you about its possibilities and the future. (As you hear about them, please don't let your own wishes and projects come in the way.)

Now it's your turn to communicate. You can express whatever you feel is of value to this being.

You may want to project towards it a wordless flow of warmth and embracing tenderness, the joy of knowing that it exists. You can transmit to it images of all that is most beautiful in this world your child will be coming into. You may communicate with music—peaceful lullabies, happy songs. You could even talk to it with words, soothing and reassuring words. The way or ways of communication are up to you.

You can continue this dialogue as long as you like, and repeat it again and again. You will thus have created the deepest relationship: the prenatal bond.

STORIES

The following stories illustrate how meaningful and powerful it is to acknowledge and connect with our babies before we can look into their eyes and hold them in our arms.

Traditional

- To ensure a safe pregnancy and avert any danger of miscarriage, the Satnami of India make a magical remedy out of a string of beads knotted ten times, which is then bound around the waist of the mother-to-be. A song is sung by the villagers to further protect the mother and unborn child. However, the string of beads must be untied before delivery to thwart off any "knots" or problems during delivery.

- In certain tribes pregnant women avoid wearing any knots at all, from their hair to their clothing, for fear that they would create "knots" in the birth.

- In most tribal societies, pregnancy creates little change for the mother. Women remain active, working in the community until the time of birth. Even then, a woman may stop her work, go to a quiet place in nature, give birth and then return to her task, carrying her newborn across her chest.

- Pregnancy care in some tribes is provided by members who are assigned to care exclusively for the mother and baby.
- In the Dagara tribe of western Africa, a ritual is performed before the baby is born that welcomes the baby's spirit into the family and affirms the parents' commitment to the child and to one another.

Personal
- When his wife was in her fifth month of pregnancy, the father of the incoming child had a dream in which he was introduced to his son, who was a young man named Caleb. The parent honored the dream as a message from their unborn child and named their son the name given to him in the dream.
- In a Nondominant Handwriting Exercise, a mother who had been experiencing uncomfortable leg cramps was advised to eliminate a certain food from her diet. When she heeded the letter's suggestion, the leg cramps vanished immediately.
- Mauris was visited by her future granddaughter, who told her to "get her mother ready," because she was coming. She was present at her granddaughter's birth one year later.

Some people believe that their children can strongly influence and attract a brother or sister to their family. My friends, Diane and Jeff, are certain of this from their own story, which I call "The Story Of Grace."

- Diane insists that their adopted son, Gabriel (read "The Story of Gabriel" in Chapter Four), is responsible for attracting their second child. When Gabriel was four, he began to talk a lot about wanting to have a little sister. Around this time, Diane and Jeff had started preparations for adopting a second child. The entire family was excited.

During that winter Diane developed flulike symptoms and fatigue. When the symptoms persisted and after a missed period, Jeff persuaded a reluctant Diane to use a home pregnancy test. Even with a positive test result, she distrusted the test's viability. After a second positive test result, Diane accepted that she was indeed pregnant, but she seriously doubted the likelihood that she would carry the baby to full term. Diane knew her reaction was shaped by her history of miscarriages. At the time it just seemed easier to dismiss the whole thing. However, in the eleventh week of pregnancy, Diane was invited to view her pregnancy from a totally different perspective. One night while sleeping, Diane was awakened by a glowing white light that seemed to rise up out of her lower body and then pulsate about ten to twelve inches above her abdomen. This glow-in-the-dark light then formed into a larger-than-life female "soul" face with violet blue eyes. Diane somehow knew this stunning energy was her unborn child. Intuitively, she asked the spirit, "Are you staying?" The image responded by saying, "I am your daughter, Grace. Yes, I am staying, and everything will be fine." Diane watched the face dissolve back into the whitish light, which then disappeared back into her body. From that moment on, Diane's experience completely changed. She woke up the next morning and knew that she would give birth to a blond-haired daughter and that her name would be Grace. Diane, Jeff, and Gabriel welcomed a daughter with blond hair and violet blue eyes, named Grace, in early autumn of that year.

Rituals, Ceremonies, and Celebrations

In their unique way, each of the following rituals exquisitely honor the mother, father/birth partner, child, and their individual soul's songs, while providing opportunities to connect more deeply as a family unit before the baby arrives.

Honoring the Mother

This ritual is inspired by one that was created for me by my dear friends and colleagues right before I moved from the East Coast to the Pacific Northwest. The gathering spoke to a vision that I'd had several months before our moving date.

In the vision I saw a Native American woman standing on the outer edge of her village. She was preparing for a journey. The time had finally come for her to travel into the vast wilderness that was before her. Sadness filled the air, yet there was a sense of celebration—for the journey, or vision quest, was one of honor. As loved ones gathered around her, they lovingly laid beautiful gifts upon a vibrantly colored woolen blanket and said their goodbyes.

Much like in my vision, on one summery evening, in the magical Berkshire mountains, my special friends came to say goodbye to me. The ceremony took place beneath one of my favorite trees, an ancient sycamore. We shared food, stories, and fond memories. Despite a visit from mosquitoes the size of minivans, this creative bunch improvised and sang a song for me, and on the blanket they laid out before me gifts for my journey. This gift bundle, imbued with their genuine love and caring, traveled with me across the country and now rests on my altar. The gift has been a lovely reminder of my special friends and the night that my soul's song was honored!

What you will need: invitations, sage or incense, candles, blanket, flowers, mother's sacred objects, musical instruments or recorded music, and gifts for the mother.

Adapting this ritual can be a gorgeous way to honor the mother-to-be. Invite your dearest friends. Send out special invitations. You can include your partner and children, or you might want to experience this ceremony with just your closest female friends. You may even ask your partner or a friend to help you organize and plan this ritual. As always, trust your instinct!

Have the gathering in a special place in your own home, a friend's home, or in a favorite place outdoors. You might think of this ceremony as creating *sacred ground* for the birth. Whether you plan for your baby to be born at home, in a birthing center, or at a hospital, surround yourself with some of the objects from this ritual. It is a way to bring the *sacred ground* with you—no matter where you give birth!

Since this ritual is *honoring the mother,* the directions are written for the facilitators of the gathering.

Purify the ceremonial space with sage or incense. Lay out a blanket. In the blanket's center create an altar with candles and a vase of flowers (roses are a beautiful symbol for this ceremony—or select the mother's favorite flowers). Ask those attending the ceremony to bring little gifts for the mother's journey (the mother's animal totem, a polished stone, a poem—anything that might be meaningful to her). Collect the gifts in a bundle, a basket, or a silk scarf. These gifts can be given as part of the ceremony after each friend shares her thoughts, well wishes, and prayers for the mother. Include saying blessings for the mother and child to have a safe journey. Everyone can then be invited to play music together. (Either have everyone bring some kind of instrument, such as a Native American drum, rattle, or recorder, or listen to a special piece of music on a compact disk or audio cassette). Get up and dance. If you are a daring group, practice with the mother making primal sounds. Many midwives believe that opening up the throat opens up the pathways for birth. It certainly can be a wonderful way to break down some of the inhibitions that so plague our culture, and help give the mother more freedom in her delivery style.

If the mother is comfortable with being touched, massage her feet, give her a back rub, wash or brush her hair, give her a sponge bath. One mother wanted her toe nails painted! She was delighted. She said it had been a long while since she had gotten a pedicure or even see her toes! The main idea here is to nurture, honor, and adorn her as she prepares for the birthing part of this remarkable journey.

Close the ceremony with a song, prayer, reading, or meditation.

Blessing Way

Deborah and Dan Howard introduced me to this ceremony—one they performed in honor of the birth of their two daughters. The ritual's origins come from the American Southwest. It is a variation of the *Honoring the Mother* ritual where women can honor women. Traditionally, the only man invited is the mother's partner.

What you will need: Invitations, sage or sweet grass, blue corn meal, bowl, pitcher of water, candles, gifts for the mother, (including her favorite food), music, and yarn for weaving a bracelet.

Purify the ceremonial space with the sage or sweet grass. Lay out a blanket. In the blanket's center create an altar with candles, flowers, gifts, and food. Have everyone sit in a circle, except for the mother who will sit or lie down in the circle's center near the altar. It is here she will be honored with loving words, touch, sound and her favorite food. She should come into the center with her hair worn up and wearing something loose and comfortable. Light a candle and talk about the purpose of the gathering. Help the mother get comfortable with pillows and a quilt. Take her hair down and brush it. (You can even wash her hair). Mix a little water into the blue corn meal and crush it into a paste, then lightly massage it into the mother's feet and hands. Rinse her feet in warm water and dry them with a soft towel. Everyone participates in cleansing, purifying, soothing, and tenderly caring for the mother and her body. You can also feed her her favorite foods and present her with special gifts and notes. Sing songs, read poetry, share stories, listen to music, laugh, cry, create moments of silence— all in honor of the mother and this sacred time. At some point, take yarn and wrap it around the mother's wrist. Continue the thread, linking each woman together, while creating a bracelet for each woman's wrist. As the yarn is tied onto a woman's wrist, she offers a prayer (which can be written down and placed in a basket for the mother to keep, or woven and tied in the bracelet). Before the close of the ceremony, cut the yarn, so that each woman can leave wearing her bracelet. The bracelet is meant to symbolize their loving connection to the mother, especially during labor and birth.

Close the ceremony with a blessing.

Mask-Making Ceremony

What you will need: sage or incense, mask-making materials (medical gauze cut in strips, bowls of water, and anything you wish to use to decorate the mask, such as paints, feathers, sequins, and pieces of fabric), elastic band and stapler (to make the strap which holds the mask onto the face), un-petroleum jelly or Vaseline (to put on the face before applying the gauze), gifts for the mother, mother's favorite food, recorded music to dance to, candles, soft blanket, cushions to sit on, flowers, pitcher of purified water, and goblets.

This ritual is inspired by Mauris Harla Justice, a health care practioner, and Hope Fay and Leah Stebbens, midwives and naturopathic physicians in Seattle, Washington, who offer this beautiful ceremony to pregnant mothers. As Fay says, "It is a wonderful time for women to come together in a circle and 'mother' the mother just as it has been done in other cultures and in other times." For this reason the ritual is designed for the pregnant woman and a female support person (her mother, sister, other family member, or a friend). Honoring the mother takes place in a group setting with other pregnant mothers and their support person. It is a lovely way to nurture, tend to, and love the new mother as she journeys from one place of being and knowing herself to another, while at the same time building and strengthening a support system and creating a new community of women friends.

There are a number of ways that you might consider doing this ritual. If you are the one pregnant, you can organize a gathering of women much like in *Honoring the Mother Ritual* or *Blessing Way* in this chapter. If you have friends who are pregnant, you can create this experience together. It will be in two parts, ideally held on different days (the masks will need to dry overnight). If the ceremony needs to be held on one day, be sure to make the masks first thing in the morning so that they can have all day to dry. Any way that you choose to use this ritual, ask your support person(s) to help you. As in any ritual or ceremony, the moment that you start preparations the healing begins.

For the ritual, select a private and intimate place. If you are planning a home birth, it is particularly powerful to do the ritual there, although it isn't necessary. (Remember you can carry the *sacred ground* with you anywhere.) Create your ceremonial space by laying out a blanket. On top of the blanket and in a circle, arrange cushions, pillows, or other blankets to sit on. Create an altar in the center of the circle with flowers, candles, and sacred objects. Also place the materials for making the masks in a basket in the center.

If this ritual is for more than one pregnant woman, ask the support-givers to bring one gift for one of the women being honored. When they arrive, have them place their gift in the center of the blanket (the altar or sacred center).

Once everyone has gathered, invite someone to light the sage or incense to purify and cleanse the space. Then light a candle on the altar. Welcome everyone and talk a little about the purpose of this gathering. This is a good time to invite everyone to share a little about herself, why she has come, what she hopes she will give and what she hopes to receive by taking part in the ritual.

Before actually making the masks, have someone lead the group in a simple guided meditation (to help everyone center themselves and relax), read a relevant passage from any favorite writing (try *A Circle of Stones: Woman's Journey to Herself,* by Judith Duerk or *Motherprayer,* by Tikva Frymer Kensky), or simply sit in silence for a few minutes.

Now the pregnant mother(s), assisted by their support person, will make the mask(s). The design of the mask should somehow express this rite of passage. Put on some music and create! Apply the un-petroleum jelly to the mother's face (to protect the skin and to help the mask come off once it is slightly dry). Dampen strips of medical gauze one at a time in a bowl of water. Then place the strips over the mother's face. Once completed let the mask set for a few minutes, and then squiggle her face around, which will help the mask come off easily. If you wish, delicately decorate the masks with paint, beads, sequins, fabric, and feathers. Lay out the mask to dry overnight (or during the course of the day while doing other activities).

When everyone is done, come back into the circle. Share your experiences. Remind everyone about meeting again. Close the ceremony with a reading, meditation, or prayer.

Before the next gathering, place the masks (now dry) in the circle's center. When everyone arrives, light the candle as before. Then invite the women to share. Did they have any dreams, thoughts, or experiences since the previous ceremony that they feel were important and/or somehow connected?

Now have each support person collect the mother's mask

from the center of the circle. Slowly and gently help the mother put on her mask. Once everyone has a mask on, sit in silence for a few moments. Look around the circle.

Put on recorded music or have everyone play some kind of musical instrument (a Native American drum, rattle, etc.) while the support people accompany the pregnant mothers as they move and dance in their masks. If you are celebrating and honoring only one mother, everyone get up and dance with her.

When this portion of the ritual is complete, return to the sitting circle. Have the mother share what the experience of moving was like for her. What was her inner self or soul expressing through the mask and through the music?

This is a perfect time to nourish and replenish the mother—pour purified water into a goblet for her to sip, feed her some of her favorite food. Tenderly massage her feet, give her a back rub or brush her hair (maybe as part of the ritual, she had her hair pulled up or back at the beginning of the ceremony). Think of truly mothering her. Take as much time as you need.

In a group experience have each pregnant woman choose one of the gifts on the altar or sacred center, and then share why she was attracted to the particular gift. Have the person who brought the gift share why she might have felt moved to bring it. If you are honoring only one mother-to-be, each person should discuss the significance of the gift given.

In closing, have someone read from meaningful text, sing together, or say a blessing of gratitude.

Communing with the Soul of the Child

What you will need: Smudge stick, sage or incense, bowl of water, candles (including a floating one if you can find one), matches, flowers, and a baby gift offering.

This lovely ritual offers a way to connect with the soul of your unborn child. You may wish to share this experience with your partner and children, or you may wish to have the experience alone. Trust your intuition. Allow your soul to guide you.

Sit in your baby's room, your *sacred space,* the *couple's sanctuary* or a favorite place outdoors. Bring a bowl of water, a floating candle, matches, flowers, and a baby offering, if you wish. The offering can be the child's *song* (with the lyrics written down), or something you have made (a poem, quilt, watercolor, an entry in your journal). If you wish, purify the space (with the smudge stick, sage or incense) before beginning the meditation.

Begin by closing your eyes. Bring your awareness to your breath. Take in a nice deep breath through your nose. Let go of that breath through your mouth, slowly and easily. Allow the breath to find its own easy and natural rhythm. Allow each breath to relax you. Each breath centering your body. Each breath easing the mind. Take as long as you need to feel relaxed and calm. Remember, at the very least, this special time is giving you and your baby a moment to rest. To be in the stillness. The quiet is so nourishing and nurturing to you both. Precious time shared together. Once you feel calm and relaxed, gently open your eyes. Light the water candle. As you do this, you might say to yourself or aloud, "May the warmth and golden light of this candle envelop this sacred space with loving guidance and wisdom." Invite your God, heavenly spirits, angels, your ancestors, the Divine—whoever you wish to assist you in this ceremony.

Looking into the flame of the floating candle, imagine your child emitting his or her golden light, safe, secure, and comfortable in the warm fluid of your womb. Allow the golden hues to flow through all of your body. Warm colors emanating out from the womb, moving, flowing, gliding through all parts of your body. Especially feel the yellow, golden, and white tones entering your heart space. Imagine the warmth flowing through and around your heart, including behind your heart. Feel the sensations.

You can either continue looking into the flame or close your eyes now. Say a blessing or prayer to the soul of the unborn. You might say something like, "I feel so blessed and thrilled about you coming into my life, I am looking forward to the time that we can hold you in our arms and look into your eyes. But for now, I honor your need to grow, unfold, and blossom in your own unique way, in your perfect time."

If you wish, sing a chant or your baby's soul song.

Now ask any questions that spontaneously arise or that you have thought of for this particular ritual. *Listen.* The responses may come through images or words, or you may experience a feeling intuitively. You may find that a response will come quickly and easily. If not, it may be helpful to do this ritual over a period of time, asking one question per ritual. Messages may clearly present themselves within the ritual ceremony or you might put your *listening* skills into action following the ritual. You never know when or how the soul will choose to communicate! (Remember my client who found his "messages" in advertising signs attached to the NYC mass transit system?). Or try any of the other baby-bonding exercises or rituals.

The following are some questions that you might ask:

- Is there anything that you would like me to know about your needs while in utero? (This could be any information related to prenatal care, such as nutrition or more self-nurturing time.)
- Is there anything that you would like me to know about the birth (e.g. choices regarding where, how, and who should be present)?
- What is our purpose of coming together?
- Why have you chosen me (or us) as your parent or family?
- What have you come to teach us?

- How can we help each other?
- What is your soul's purpose?
- How can I (we) help you work toward fulfilling this purpose?

Once you have asked the questions you wish to ask, express gratitude and thanks. Make an offering of your gift. Talk a little about the gift's significance. Place it near the candle. In a closing prayer, articulate that although this ritual is coming to a close, the candle's warm and golden light will continue to surround you and your baby throughout your journey together, especially now. You can invite the soul of the child to communicate with you at any time during the pregnancy. Close the ritual with a blessing of gratitude.

Birth Prayer Ritual

I have adapted this ritual from my friends, Ken and Marilynn, who created a sacred ceremony two months before Marilynn's due date, with friends whom they believed would be significant and special in their son's life. I think their idea beautifully and symbolically expresses the spiritual dimension of birthing a child, including involving friends and family.

You will need: Invitations, musical instruments (including a drum), candles, and matches. Read further for ideas on what materials will be needed, depending on how you choose to make the birth canal and a prayer braid.

Invite your guests to bring a musical instrument for the birthing ceremony, and food to share as part of the celebration.

The idea is to dramatize birth. Set up a symbolic womb and birth canal using streamers, scarves, empty boxes, or human bodies, either before your guests arrive or as part of the ceremony. Whatever you decide, design it so that you and your friends have to either walk or crawl through it as a way to enter the ceremonial space. Lighted candles and drumming can add to the ambiance and, in fact, help produce an overall tone of sacredness to the ceremony. Drumming also beautifully simulates the heartbeat of the mother. After you and your partner have passed through the canal first, sit down. This is a good time to begin drumming, if you wish. As your guests enter the inner ceremonial space from the birth canal, have them join you (making a circle) and they, too, can drum or play any other instrument, such as a tambourine, rattle, etc. After playing together for a few minutes, or however long you feel moved to do so, stop and welcome everyone. Express what your intention is for the gathering. For example, talk about what it means to be sharing this extraordinary time, of birthing this child, with dear friends; that together you will be honoring the birth of your child with prayers and blessings and that you see how everyone gathered is a midwife to this event. You can also talk about how giving birth is symbolic of giving birth to an ever-growing and expanding state of awareness and consciousness. You can either read words that you have written for this occasion, or select lyrics, poetry, or prose that expresses the sacredness of this time.

Invite your loved ones, one by one, to share their feelings, stories, prayers, and blessings, either silently or out loud, while they weave colored thread into a braid of yarn, or string beads onto a necklace that you have started, or tie a knot in a stretch of nylon climbing rope. As they do so, imagine each prayer, blessing, and feeling of love and support woven into the braid placed into the bead or knotted into the rope. Pass the prayer braid, necklace, or rope onto the next person. When everyone is done, including both partners, tie the braided yarn, the beaded necklace, or nylon rope into a circle. This is to be hung over the baby's crib or somewhere else in the baby's room (of course, safe from exploring little fingers); now imbued with love and prayers, it is meant to envelop and protect the child throughout his or her life. Conclude the ceremony with wonderful food and drink and more music.

*   *   *

Here are some other ideas:

- Ken and Marilynn passed around two long nylon climbing ropes with different colors. As the ropes came around the circle, each person said a prayer (silently or out loud) and tied a knot into each rope. Ken and Marilynn purposefully guided the ropes behind each person (after the prayer knots were tied) symbolizing how the entire community was included in the birthing of this child. One prayer rope was to be left in their baby's room; the other rope was cut apart at the close of the ceremony. Everyone was then invited to take a knot (containing one of the prayers offered in the ceremony) home with them. Ken and Marilynn's idea was that each person would then become a "Keeper of the Prayer"—safely keeping and holding close the prayers and blessings offered to their unborn child. The knots also symbolically expressed how "tied" together they all were as a family and a community.
- At the end of the ritual, everyone was invited to paint Marilynn's wonderfully round belly. They had so much fun doing this that they spontaneously turned to each other and began to paint one another's faces. In the process of the ritual, a child was lovingly welcomed with intimate prayers and blessings, and a tribe was born!
- Have your loved ones say their prayer as they weave a piece of greenery or fresh or dried flowers into a circular or heart-shaped wire mesh form, creating a wreath.
- Make a bracelet or necklace out of yarn and/or beads.
- Pass around a large, round sheet of heavy-stock white paper and a basket full of colored pens, pencils, or crayons. Create a mandala together (a mandala is a sacred circular healing symbol).
- Make a collage. Pass around a basket of scissors, glue,

fabric swatches, ribbon, photographs, pictures from magazines, or whatever else you have gathered (you could even invite your guests to bring something for this purpose). After offering their prayer, have your guests select something from the basket and glue it on a piece of poster board cut in an egg shape, or whatever other shape you feel works best for this purpose.

The beauty of this ceremony, as in any other, is to make it uniquely yours. Remember to place the symbol, imbued with love and care, somewhere safe in your baby's room. Envision the prayers and blessings unfolding, growing, and blossoming, right alongside your child.

Ode to Birth

This ritual is designed for the mother and her partner as preparation for the birthing experience. It includes a beautiful meditation from *The Child of Your Dreams,* by Huxley and Ferrucci, which can also be practiced as an exercise all by itself.

You will need: smudge stick or incense, a candle, rose or lavender water mist, flowers, pens, pencils or paints, art pad or your journal, and sacred objects (anything that holds special meaning for you, or something given to you or your baby during another ceremony, such as a prayer braid). For the mother you also might want to bring extra pillows (for extra comfort, especially toward the end of pregnancy).

In your sacred space, shared sanctuary or, if having a home birth, the place you will be giving birth, sit comfortably. If you wish, lightly smudge the space and then mist it with rose or lavender water. Light a candle. Focus on your breath. Allow your breath to center and ground you. In your mind or out loud, state the purpose of this ritual and then begin the *Birth Date Meditation.*

BIRTH DATE MEDITATION

The birth of your baby is coming. You are counting the days now. The following meditation is helpful to generate a beautiful atmosphere for your baby; to help you, the mother, to be more serene and relaxed; and also you, the father, to participate in this memorable event.

Lie down, and for a long while, as long as it feels comfortable, just breathe.

Breathe deeply and slowly. Imagine that all cares, all tensions, all preconceived notions of birth, in fact all thoughts, are leaving you with each exhalation. Imagine that the air, rather than coming in and out through the nose or mouth, is penetrating you through the whole surface of your body: the entire surface of your skin has become your breathing organ. Take a lot of time to learn to breathe in this new way. Without forcing, let your breathing become deeper and deeper.

As you breathe with your whole body, become aware of the air you breathe. Feel, imagine, that this air is vibrating with vital energy—that it penetrates everywhere in your body: where you are tired, it regenerates you; where you are tense, it relaxes you; where you feel empty, it fills you with light and life.

Now you are going to create the environment in which you want to welcome the baby into the world. Where would you like your child to be born?

near the ocean, amidst the shells and the splashes and the
   balmy
smell of the sea . . .
at night, pervaded by silence, under the stars . . .
under a giant oak, feeling its ancient strength . . .
during spring, in the midst of a meadow full of flowers
   of
all colors
In ripe wheat, experiencing the fertility and richness

of the earth . . .
under a gentle rain or a rainbow . . .

near a waterfall . . .
on the mountains, surrounded by pure, crisp mountain
    air . . .
at dawn or sunset.

These are just a few examples. It is up to you to imagine the environment you prefer. Whatever the setting you have chosen, visualize it as clearly as you can. Imagine actually being there. Breathe in, feel the smell, the tactile sensations, hear the sounds, and see the colors vividly. As you repeat this exercise, images will become more alive and richer, so do not be discouraged if you do not succeed at first. By visualizing the same setting again and again, you will make it more and more alive. Whatever your outer environment will be, within the vast space of your mind and through the resources of your imagination, you will actually be creating a living reality in your inner world—and in the inner world of your baby.

Imagine your baby is there with you, newly born. Communicate with your baby with words or songs or through your skin. Talk to him or her about this new world he/she is being born into. Surround your baby with a tender, loving welcome.

As you open your eyes, and slowly, very slowly, come back to everyday consciousness, draw or paint the setting you have chosen for your child to be born in. Remember, perfection and style have no relevance here. Just express in any way that is easy to you the feelings and the images you have had during this meditation.

Complete the ritual by expressing gratitude. Put your drawing/painting on your altar or somewhere where you can see it often.

Singing the Child's Song

You will need: Lavender or rose water mist, matches, candles (or build a campfire outdoors or a fire in a fireplace), flowers, a basket of small white tapered candles, a variety of musical instruments, or a selection of recorded music.

The intention of this ritual is to honor the unborn child by acknowledging and honoring her *song*. Perhaps through this ceremony you will hear your child's *song* for the first time, or maybe you already have a sense of what it is. Just remember that the soul's song can not only be a literal *song* but also a poem, a story, a piece of prose, a chant, a dance, or a meditation. It may even be the child's name. This ritual offers a sacred place and a sacred way to honor your child's unique beingness.

You can either perform this ritual alone or use it as a way to introduce your child and teach his or her *song* to loved ones—especially those who will be present at the physical birth.

In your sacred space, couple's sanctuary, a special place in nature, or anywhere else that is meaningful to you, sit quietly. Use an aromatherapy diffuser or spray a mist of rose oil mixed in water. If you are outdoors, make a campfire; if you are indoors, light a candle, a fire in a fireplace or use a wood-burning stove as your centerpiece. In an opening prayer, express the intention of this ceremony—"We come together to honor the spirit and soul of (name of baby, if you have chosen a name). We invite and welcome this being lovingly into our world, into our lives, and into our hearts." Imagine your prayer rising up toward the heavens on the flame and smoke of the candle or firelight.

If you feel as though you already know your child's *song,* introduce it to those gathered. Share how it came to you and what it means. Then you can either "perform" the *song* or teach the *song* to those attending so that you can sing it together. (You can think of it as a rehearsal for the child's birth!) Read, together and/or separately, meaningful words you have selected from a poem or story, or hum, chant or sing in unison. Play a piece of music and dance. Welcome the soul of the child as a celebration!

If you feel as though the *song* is still eluding you, invite everyone gathered to sit quietly in a circle. State that you are open to listening to the voice or special *song* of the child forthcoming, that you hold this space as sacred ground for her coming. Just by acknowledging that the child has her very own exquisite *song* (without necessarily identifying it) honors her soul.

Drum or play music together for a while, if you wish. Then, pass around a basket of small tapered candles. White candles are always nice, but allow your intuition to guide you. Perhaps the incoming spirit has a color preference!

As each person lights a candle, ask them to offer a prayer or blessing for this child, or share how they are feeling about her coming. They may do this silently or out loud. Once everyone has lighted a candle and shared, continue sitting together in the circle silently.

Conclude the ceremony with a favorite song, poem, or selection from prose. Or read something that you have composed especially for this gathering. Assure the soul that you will keep listening for her soul's *song,* or any other messages, but most importantly that you welcome and celebrate her presence in your life.

4

Welcoming

BIRTH

On the day you were born
the Earth turned, the moon pulled
the Sun flared, and, then, with a push,
you slipped out of the dark quiet
where suddenly you could hear . . .
. . . a circle of people singing
with voices familiar and clear.

"Welcome to the spinning world," the people sang
as they washed your new, tiny hands.
"Welcome to the green Earth," the people sang,
as they wrapped your wet, slippery body.
And as they held you close
they whispered into your open, curving ear,
"We are so glad you've come!"

DEBRA FRASIER
"On The Day You Were Born"

As I sat down to write this chapter, I found myself feeling overwhelmed—utterly daunted by the task at hand. Where do I begin? There are so many decisions that need to be considered and made as we prepare for the birth of our child. I wondered, "How do I properly guide this special reader in the most helpful way?"

I painstakingly began to look over every question and every bit of information that I had gathered. Then it dawned on me. Of course I was feeling overwhelmed. I was in labor! I began to think that birthing a first book was similar to a mother birthing her first baby in one major way. And that is that neither of us (or probably most women) has ever had the opportunity to observe or assist another women giving birth. This is unlike women in traditional cultures, who as young girls are taught about birth from the older women in their communities, including their mothers. Birth in these societies is considered a normal and natural experience of community life, an event to be participated in by all.

"In the past, having a baby was accepted as a natural event, a part of nature, like the flow of the tides and the phases of the moon," says Gina Maria Alibrandi, mother of three children, childbirth educator, and R.N. "Birth was a part of everyone's developmental experience, as people had large families and young women gave birth in their home or in the home of another family member. . . . A woman pregnant for the first time already had secondhand experience of the ebb and flow of labor. She knew that she should expect arduous work and that labor would probably hurt. She also knew that she could count on the support of the women in her community to provide her with massage, hot and cold compresses, herbal teas, and other comfort measures when her time came to embark on the journey of motherhood. . . .the birth of a baby was a joyous event, accompanied by great celebration and tremendous pride felt by the entire extended family and community." *(Trust Your Body! Trust Your Baby!,* edited by Andrea Frank Henkart).

Since most of us no longer have the opportunity to be taught by wise women elders or to assist in the births of family and community members, we need to find other ways to re-learn how to give birth to our babies.

Midwives and women working as doulas (birth assistants) are doing superb work in helping women in the western world reclaim their natural ability and confidence to birth their babies in the manner in which they choose. In fact, recent research shows that childbirth goes more smoothly and that mothers bond more easily with their newborns following a birth assisted by a doula.

Many women whose first child may have been born in a hospital setting—with drugs, and perhaps an unplanned caesarian—have dramatically transformed their next birth experience, with the support and nurturing care of a midwife and/or doula. They have had extraordinary and meaningful experiences giving birth at home and in birthing centers, where they have the freedom to walk, be massaged, soak in warm water while being surrounded by their family (including their children, if they wish) and friends. They squat, get down on their hands and knees, moan, cry, and are held by their birth partners as their baby emerges into our world.

The nurse who taught Tracy's childbirth class warned her that she would be told not to make any noise when she was ready to bear down to push—that the current theory was that it would cause the baby to "slip back"—and that's exactly what happened. Fortunately, in the throes of labor the need to grunt was greater than her inclination to be a "good patient," and Tracy told her doctor that she wanted to try it her way first. Now pregnant with her second baby and under the care of a different ob-gyn, she plans to moan and groan without apology when she gives birth this summer.

Anna recently gave birth to her first baby in a birthing room. Along with her obstetrician, her insurance policy allowed for a midwife to work with her throughout her pregnancy. Anna was impressed at how knowledgeable her midwife was about the medical/technological as well as the natural aspects of giving birth. The midwife, obstetrician, and Anna's husband, Steve, together assisted mother and child in the birthing process. And even though the birth ended up being a caesarian, due to several complications, Anna felt that she and her baby were tenderly cared for and honored throughout the entire experience.

Another friend gave birth to her second daughter (her first was delivered by caesarian) while being cradled by her husband in a birthing tub in a beautiful birthing center with a doula and obstetrician assisting.

Leslie is so grateful for the wonderful support that she received from her midwife and doula during the pregnancy and birth of her second son, Larkin, she became trained as a doula and teaches a course on counseling at a midwifery school.

Modern childbirth education is making an excellent effort to replace some of the lost traditional practices of teaching and learning about birthing babies. Classes with professionals trained and experienced in childbirth, as well as viewing videos, can provide very important information. Insightful doctors, such as Grantly Dick-Read, Ferdinand Lamaze, and Robert Bradley, introduced their respective childbirth approaches based on the crucial role breathing plays in pain relief, which began to help and encourage women to return to their own natural abilities to birth their babies. Their approaches, along with self-hypnosis, visualization, and other relaxation techniques have been helpful to many women during childbirth.

However, the most integral element of childbirth that has been lost in our culture is the way women have become disconnected from trusting the innate wisdom and power of their bodies. With the advancements in medicine, especially in obstetrics, we have somehow been convinced that we need medical intervention in order to deliver our babies safely. We can certainly be grateful for what modern medicine offers. An intervention skillfully and appropriately administered may influence a mother's and/or baby's physical well-being, even their survival. The question is, how often are these interventions used unnecessarily?

Since the 1970's obstetricians Frederick Leboyer (*Birth*

Without Violence) and Michel Odent (*Birth Reborn*) have been passionate about helping women birth their babies with less obstetrics and more in the way that feels natural and instinctual.

The uterus, the cervix, the vagina, the heart, the lungs—our whole body knows what to do to give birth. The human body is truly a miracle. However, women in our culture are not generally taught, inspired, or supported to trust in the perfection of their bodies and to have faith in their abilities to birth their children. When we are allowed to birth our babies the way that feels true and natural, we spontaneously connect to the wisdom and miracle of our bodies. In reconnecting with this part, we know how to care for ourselves during all of the stages of birthing a child, including riding the dramatic and painful waves of labor and birth with more ease and confidence. Trusting our body, mind, and heart opens us more fully to the journey that brings our babies into our lives.

Another element sadly missing in our childbirth practices is honoring that our babies carry within them their own wisdom and that they have a consciousness from the very beginning; that they, too, are capable of feeling fear, anger, and joy. And that they perceive and feel our feelings as well.

Tragically, our misguided beliefs and lack of awareness have resulted in the establishment of birthing practices that are not only insensitive to mother and baby at birth, but may cause lifelong harm to the developing child. Recent studies are finding correlations between the dramatic rise in violence in our culture and the nature of our prenatal and birth practices. (See *Recommended Reading* and *Resources* for more on the subject of babies having an awareness, beginning in the womb).

In the words of Suzanne Arms, the provocative and passionate author of *Immaculate Deception* and *Immaculate Deception II,* "The real purpose of childbirth education ought to be helping people prepare for the coming of a new soul. We must do whatever we can to open our hearts and adjust our circumstances to fit the need and pace of this human being for whom every experience will be fresh, and who will be completely dependent on us. Lifelong trust is established by how safe and wanted we feel at the beginning of life."

Many traditional cultures honor the notion that our children come into our lives awake, aware, and with a purpose. Anne Hubbell Maiden, Ph.D., has discovered in studying numerous traditional cultures that there are certain similarities in birth practices which reflect these beliefs, including: dialoguing with the unborn, the unity of the birthing family and community, a reverence for life, a respect and love for the earth, purposeful rituals, welcoming ceremonies, massage and touch, the importance of dreams, expressing gratitude, seeing birth as a natural passage, establishing sacred family time, honoring the realm of spirit and the inherent mystery of life and belief that all beings have a life purpose.

A wonderful question to ponder is how can these elements inspire, teach, motivate, and encourage us to create and enrich our own practices, customs, and traditions for welcoming our children? How can we truly honor their soul's song throughout the birthing experience?

Many of us approach childbirth naively. In a culture that doesn't easily or naturally respect women's inner wisdom and knowledge, we (unconsciously and consciously) have relinquished our trust in ourselves to the "experts."

Of all the women I have talked to about their birth story, a large number of those who gave birth in a conventional hospital setting expressed feelings of guilt, shame, frustration, and anger about their birth experiences. Women who had caesarians felt especially guilty and ashamed—because they carry the belief that they somehow had failed. Yet, whether they delivered vaginally or surgically, the overall experience left them feeling dazed and perplexed, if not in shock. One friend found herself in a severe postpartum depression. Another friend who had birthed her baby vaginally spoke of how odd and disconnected she felt from all of her friends, who had delivered their babies by cesareans. Although everyone ended up with beautiful and healthy babies, she felt extremely alone in her experience. Most women commented on how "hungry" they had been to hear other women's birth stories, as well as to tell their own. Listening and sharing seemed to help them appreciate their own birth experience, and the gamut of feelings that were birthed right along with their baby.

Before gathering the stories for this book, I honestly only knew a few women who had what they called a positive and joyful birth experience. For most of us, we have relegated our "unpleasant", "painful", "disappointing" experiences to secret places within. For many women, that secret place is in our female heart—the womb.

AN OCEAN OF TEARS

I was overjoyed when we returned upstate to our farm house. Crossing the threshold, this time with Zach in my arms rather than inside my belly, marked a new and exciting rite of passage. However, I found myself drenched in tears, off and on for several weeks. Zach continued to cry as well. Was I experiencing postpartum depression? Hormonal Hell? Was Zach's inconsolable crying a gastrointestinal problem? Or was he allergic to my milk? A sympathetic pediatrician said it was "colic" (a diagnosis often given when there is no other way to explain a baby's inconsolable crying spells). What I'm more likely to believe is that our ocean of tears was the work of our souls, cleansing and purifying as we began or continued the intricate weaving of our soul's journey.

Deep tissue massage, osteopathy, hypnotherapy, acupuncture, visualization, art therapy, and psychodrama are some of the approaches that can be extremely helpful in our healing efforts around birth. There are even professionals trained specifically in healing birth trauma, who are doing phenomenal work with their patients of all ages (see *Resources*). The following story conveys how essential the father or birth partner (who can typically feel left out and disconnected from mother and baby throughout the pregnancy and birth) is to the birthing experience and how transformative this type of healing work can be.

DANIEL

Hope (a naturopathic physician and midwife trained in Birth Trauma Healing Work) and one of the families with whom she worked generously shared the following story.

A couple who had just recently given birth to their first child, Daniel, made an appointment with Hope to see if she could help them. The problem was that every time the father held his new son, the baby would scream and cry hysterically. This, of course, distressed everyone.

Hope had asked the parents to tell her the story of their son's birth, and the father revealed that he had never felt connected to this baby. He also shared that as a kind of joke, he would sometimes refer to his son as his "little yuppie toy." And the entire time he is speaking to Hope, the baby boy is crying intensely, arching his back and trying his hardest not to allow his father to hold him.

But then a remarkable thing happened. The father recalled that when their doctor had put the newborn into his arms and asked, "Well, how does it feel?" he had replied, "He doesn't feel like mine." Hearing his own words for the first time, he turned to his distraught son, looked directly into his tear-filled infant eyes and lovingly said, "Oh, I'm so sorry. Daniel, I love you very much. I am so happy that you are here in my life. I love you!"

Guess what? Daniel stopped crying, his body began to relax, and he looked right back into his father's eyes. The father tenderly picked his son up, kissed him on his forehead, and held him as he never had held him before. In that instant the "issue" vanished.

This is a poignant example of how awake and aware our babies are and how sensitive they are both to their birth experience and to the attitudes, beliefs, and emotions (however subtle) of their parents. It also demonstrates how, when parents are open to growing and healing, the results can be life-transforming, for them and most especially for the child.

If you have had an unhappy, disappointing, or painful birthing experience, use those feelings as the perfect catalyst for healing (see *Grieving Loss, Welcoming the Soul of a Child Healing Ritual*) and/or clarifying and asserting what your needs and wishes are for the next birth experience. We certainly can all be a support and advocate for other future mothers and babies. As we educate and support ourselves and one another, we honor ourselves, our babies, our babies' babies, and so on. In reclaiming our innate wisdom and power to birth our babies in the way that best fits our beliefs, we are then able to pass on an astounding lineage—one that began millions of years ago. Pain always has the potential for birthing passionate action. Together we can become a dynamic force, instrumental in transforming not only the way we birth our babies, but the way we consciously welcome and honor our children throughout all of their lives.

FATHERS

It is my hope that as women begin to reclaim their innate wisdom and authority, especially when it comes to birthing their children, that fathers, too, will discover and create a deeper connection to the overall birth experience. As my male friends and husband remind me, men often feel separate and left out. Just given the nature of anatomy, it is understandable why men feel this way. After all, the baby is growing inside the mother's body, and it will be her body from which the baby will emerge. No one would argue that conceiving, carrying, and birthing a baby is anything less than a miraculous rite of passage for women, awe-inspiring and powerful. Yet, as we are learning, the father's presence has a significant impact. We know that the way in which he supports, assists, loves, and honors his partner does transmit to the unborn child. Yet, often the quality and quantity of his support is directly related to the degree to which he feels connected, physically, mentally, and spiritually, to the whole experience.

Interestingly, some indigenous cultures, for various reasons, send the father away when his wife becomes pregnant and/or when she is birthing their child. The mother may be cared for exclusively by her own family or other female elders, who will help her birth the baby. However, in most indigenous societies, the father is integral to the birthing experience, beginning before conception.

The Aborigines believe that the spirit of a child appears in the father's dreams or inner awareness before conception. Among the Basque people in the Pyrenees, both mother and father-to-be will dialogue with the unborn baby—telling it stories about their life together. Together they also sing songs that will be repeated during and after the birth. In the Tibetan culture, the father recites periodically from a collection of mantras throughout the birth experience. And with the help of the dukun (healer) and a female relative, he will also "catch" the baby. Before the cord is cut, he will be the one to recite the traditional prayers. In Bali, fathers share in childrearing, carrying the children everywhere while talking to them one on one.

We, as a culture, have made progress since the days when fathers were either sent to fetch the proverbial pot of boiling water or directed to the hospital's waiting room to wait with other fathers-to-be, while their child was "being delivered."

However, we still need to cultivate customs and traditions that truly honor and respect the mother, child, and father. Fortunately, courageous visionaries and pioneers in the field of childbirth, including mothers and fathers who are becoming more vocal about how they want their child to be born, are beginning to transform the way that we bring our children into the world.

Fathers, as you travel the path of becoming a parent, I encourage you and your partner to *birth* your own practices, customs, and traditions to strengthen your feeling of connection. All the stages of bringing a baby into our world invite us to grow and deepen individually and as a couple. Refer to the *Index of Exercises and Rituals* for opportunities that can help facilitate a more meaningful connection. Also read the following section on Water Births, which describes how participating in aqua-natal classes beautifully fosters closeness.

WATER BIRTHS

We Are All Water Babies is a breathtaking book by Jessica Johnson and Michel Odent. Odent, a world famous obstetrician, observed that women were naturally drawn to water during labor, and decided one day to bring an inflatable blue paddling pool to the maternity hospital where he worked in Pithiviers, France. In the thirty-some years since then, Odent has brilliantly inspired the way for creating birthing practices that are gentler, more supportive, and more respectful for both mother and child. Johnson, a gifted underwater photographer, wanted to illustrate the link that water provides in our lives from birth to death. Their collaboration makes *We Are All Babies* a provocative journey into the healing powers of water.

First, the photographs are utterly captivating! Many depict parents and their babies (five weeks and up) learning how to swim with Lauren Heston, a gifted teacher who specializes in baby/child/parent swimming classes, in Pithiviers, France. These exquisite underwater pictures of cherubic babies gliding through the water, eyes open, reflect how these little creatures show no fear when first introduced to the water (in trained hands, of course!). The text, equally engaging, tells of studies done on babies who learn to swim early on and how it has helped to enhance their unfolding in a myriad of ways (socially, physically, emotionally, and intellectually).

The book also describes the work of Dr. Herman Ponette, who, after visiting Odent in France, returned to his home in Ostend, Belgium, and began developing water birth practices. Dr. Ponette has helped over 2,000 women birth their babies. The hospital in Ostend uses a specially designed birthing tub and with the use of mirrors, birthing mothers can watch their babies emerge from their bodies.

A unique aspect of his program is the aqua-natal classes, run by a group called Aquarius. These classes create a remarkable opportunity for the woman and her partner to bond with each other and with the child during pregnancy and in preparation for childbirth. Many pregnant couples find swimming together a good way to relieve everyday stress, all the while strengthening the women's bodies for giving birth. During labor, both mother and partner are in the water doing many of the breathing and movement exercises they practiced in class. In the first weeks of their baby's life, parents return to the warm water with their newborn. With the guidance and encouragement of skilled instructors, the new families swim together. The element of water offers a continuum, a satin thread that deeply bonds parents and child.

What I think is particularly wonderful is how this style of birthing—especially the swimming classes—fosters more involvement and participation by the father. Adapting and incorporating the birthing practices modeled by Odent and Ponette, especially the aqua-natal classes, can provide an excellent way for the father to feel more bonded to mother and baby, as well as to have a central role in his child's birth. Ultimately, using water as the medium to welcome, bond, and nurture our children fosters opportunity for both parents to deeply connect to one another and to their child. It is a model that superbly integrates body, mind, heart, and soul (of parents and child) during one of life's most magnificent rites of passage.

More and more couples are asking for warm water immersion during labor and/or the birth. Water births have been practiced in many indigenous cultures for thousands of years, and studies reflect the fact that over 50,000 water births have taken place in the world over the last ten years, with no reports of life-threatening complications for either mother or baby. In the United States there are approximately 140 hospitals or birth centers that have portable pools or permanent pools for the purpose of water labor and/or birth.

Water births are not for everyone, but if you find yourself drawn to this model, you can contact the Global Maternal/Child Health Association for the most current information on the subject. Their address is listed in *Resources,* along with information about childbirth education, midwife and doula groups and organizations.

Ultimately, there are all kinds of ways to bring a baby into our world. There is not one perfect or magical way. Each woman, each baby, each situation is exquisitely unique. What makes one woman feel confident and safe may create entirely different feelings for someone else. For example, for some women, having a home birth would generate tremendous anxiety, for another it might provide the safest and most comfortable environment. It is extremely important to gather all of the information regarding the myriad of birthing options available, so you can make the choices that feel right for you. And, at some point in the process, always include tuning into your own intuition and inner wisdom as well as your baby's, for guidance.

(See *Index for Exercises and Rituals* to help you access this wisdom).

One of the most important values of participating in exercises, rituals, and ceremonies throughout this precious time, is to build upon the more classical approach to childbirth while reawakening and reviving the heart and soul dimension of bringing forth children into the world.

The moment of birth is a dynamic electromagnetic dance, a brilliantly played symphony—an exquisite blending of the most powerful elements of nature and life's mysteries. When a newborn travels from some unknown world to this earthly plane, we cannot help but be moved to the core of our being when he arrives and gazes into our eyes for the first time.

Cultivating Skills

All of the skills that you have been introduced to and are practicing will have tremendous importance to you and your baby as you prepare for the physical birth. *Being Present, Self-Nurturing, Strengthening the Relationship, Dialoguing, Creative Journaling, Listening, Healing Grief, Forgiveness, Baby Bonding, Communing with the Soul of the Child, Visualization,* and *Sense Awareness* all help to facilitate and access the wellspring of knowledge, guidance, strength, and compassion that resides within you. *The Reservoir* offers a way to access the boundless wealth of your inner and outer resources.

The Reservoir

Being clear on what we need and then asking for support is another important skill to cultivate. You might think of it as "calling forth" the resources around you. That is what the *Birth Plan* is all about. Invite only those people into your birthing experience who you feel will respect, support, and honor you and your baby during the birthing journey. When

I speak about bringing the *sacred ground* (the *sacred space* on wheels—sacred items from your altar, the *Prayer Braid, Baby Bundle,* a special blanket, flowers, music, or whatever else you feel is meaningful) into the birthing place, that includes the individuals you wish to be there.

Following the birth, many indigenous cultures establish "sacred family time," in which the new mother, baby, and sometimes the entire family, are doted upon and cared for by the community. This gives the mother the opportunity to rest and renew, while adjusting to the baby's rhythms and needs. In France and Sweden, mothers are given maternity leave with full pay for one and two years, respectively. In Holland, home care nursing is provided in the first several months to help the mother not only with the baby, but marketing, cooking, and cleaning.

Unfortunately for many of us, we live in a culture where once the baby is born, we are rushed out of the hospital, hurried home, and then expected to hustle back to work. We are often separated from our extended families (a possible source of support), if not geographically, then by life-styles that do not allow time for lending hands and hearts. During a time when we should be "drinking in the sweetness and love that a new-born brings to the world" (Suzanne Arms), we are thrust back into the frantic pace of our lives.

One place to begin to create nurturing after-birth care is to ask your friends and family to help out with shopping, cooking, cleaning, doing errands, taking care of your other children, or watching the baby so that you can take a shower or a walk, especially in the first several weeks. You can also hire a postpartum doula, who specializes in helping you and the baby in any way needed. In the Northwest, families find support from a nonprofit-social service organization based in Seattle called PEPS (Program For Early Parent Support); weekly, facilitated meetings with other new parents offer encouragement and a sense of connection to others who are faced with similar challenges. (See *Resources* for more information on support for new parents).

Asking for support is actually a wonderful practice in receiving. Give yourself, your baby, and the family the luxury of adjusting, resting, and bonding—nourishing elements that endure for a lifetime.

By "calling forth" from the lush and rich *reservoir* the resources that dwell within or those that exist around us, we strengthen, deepen, and grow—providing the perfect net to lovingly catch our babies as they soar into our world.

EXERCISES

As we prepare for the birth of our child, it is essential to explore our feelings. Embracing the entire range of our feelings begins to dissolve the armor that can distance us from this extraordinary rite of passage as well as from connecting with our newborn child. *Dialoguing with Fear, Exploring and Changing Your Beliefs about Birth, Birthing Mantra, The Blossoming Flower* and *Birth Energy Meditation* offer meaningful and effective ways to support you and your baby during the momentous event of labor and birth.

Dialoguing with Fear

Dialoguing facilitates communication between ourselves and that which we need to better understand—be it a physical symptom, a person, a situation, or a specific emotion. Fear is a common feeling experienced during this dramatic time of change. Through the process of *dialoguing,* however, you can explore, illuminate and process an emotion that can otherwise interfere with your and your baby's well-being. (Remember, you can substitute any feeling into this exercise.)

* * *

In your sacred space, light a candle and sit comfortably. Close your eyes and focus on your breath. Allow the breath to center and ground you. Take as long as you need to feel relaxed and still. When ready, get in touch with your fear. Notice how you feel the fear in your body, in your mind. . . . Then invite the fear to appear. Simply allow any images, thoughts, or feelings to present themself. When the fear appears, spend a few moments noticing everything about it. Where you feel it in your body is a good place to start. What color is the fear? What shape does it take or feel like? Then ask the fear to talk to you in a way that you can understand. What is it trying to communicate to you? As you sit quietly, notice if any bodily sensations arise, these are a wonderful way to receive messages from within. You can ask your fear if it is residing anywhere in your body right now. If you get a strong sensation in any particular part of your body, bring your attention fully there. Ask that part of your body what it wishes to say in words. (Remember the response may come immediately or some other time. Responses may also come to you not as words but as a visual image, a "gut feeling," or an intuitive insight.)

Ask what you can do to help ease, diminish, or release the fear. For example, you may have tremendous fear about labor and birth. If this is your first birth experience, maybe you have concerns that something will go wrong or that you won't be able to birth your baby the "right way," and you notice that the fear is manifesting itself as tightness in your shoulders. Ask the tightness or the fear what it is wanting to say to you in words. Perhaps the fear replies that, "I am the pressure that you are putting on yourself to do all of this (the pregnancy and birth) 'perfectly.' Next, ask your fear how you can transform it into something more helpful to you and your baby. Your fear might suggest practicing one of the Birth Visualizations *(The*

Blossoming Flower or *Birth Energy Meditation)* or working with a hypnotherapist who specializes in childbirth. Write and/or draw in your journal what you learn.

In any *dialoguing* exercise, first connect with the feeling that you are working on (fear, anger, grief), do a body scan, and locate where you express or hold this feeling in your body. Then ask the feeling or body sensation what it wants to communicate to you in words, and what you can do to help diminish or transform that feeling into something more helpful.

Exploring and Changing Your Beliefs About Birth

This exercise comes from *Creating a Joyful Birth Experience* by Lucia Capacchione and Sandra Bardsley. The purpose of the exercise is to identify and transform some of your unconscious and conscious beliefs about birthing a child.

Take out a sheet of paper and divide it in half. At the top of the left-hand side, write Beliefs About Labor And Delivery. On the right-hand side, write Origin Of Belief.

With your dominant hand, write your beliefs about labor and delivery in the left-hand column. It is very important to try not to think too much about this, just write the first things that come to mind. When you're finished, switch your pen or pencil to your nondominant hand, and on the right-hand side, begin writing where each belief came from. Writing and then seeing these beliefs in print can be quite revealing. Take a few moments to reflect on where these beliefs might have originated, and how they affect you negatively and positively. Once you have done this take out another sheet of paper and, with your nondominant hand, list the beliefs that you wish to keep. Think of creating new beliefs as well.

Birthing Mantra

As a student of meditation for over twenty years, I found this exercise in *Mind Over Labor,* by Carl Jones, really appealing. I have discovered the mantra is a wonderful technique for focusing, as well as offering the healing benefits of sound and vibration. Some women have found using a mantra during labor particularly helpful for creating a more relaxed state, both physically and mentally, while reducing the sense of fear and pain.

USING MANTRA

This is a simple version of the famous Eastern meditation technique of using mantra—the repetitive incantation of a sound or sounds.

Get into a comfortable position.

Allow your breathing to become a little deeper and a little slower without straining in any way.

Then repeat the same word over and over, either silently or softly as you exhale. A long, drawn-out OM ("Oohhmmm") is traditionally used. You might want to try the word "baby." As you repeat your chosen word, let yourself drift into a deeper, more relaxed state.

One day in one of my meditation sessions, the word "Love" appeared. I spontaneously began to repeat the word out loud and then to myself. It has since become my mantra. I suggest that you experiment with different sounds and words. If you *listen* maybe your baby will whisper or sing a mantra into your ear that will help carry you both on the natural waves, rhythms, and sounds of birth.

Birthing Visualization

The following visualization is also one that Carl Jones uses. It can be found in his book, *Visualizations for an Easier Child-*

birth. Many have found that this imagery is easy to connect to, thus very effective during the rigors of labor.

THE BLOSSOMING FLOWER

An opening flower is the perfect symbol for both the opening cervix and the widening vagina. No image better captures the qualities of warmth, beauty, softening, moisture, fragrance, and opening. (Jones observes that the vagina is often referred to as a flower in the ancient poetry of India and China).

This very simple, lovely exercise is the most popular for labor and one of the most effective. Use it any time during your labor, with or between contractions.

Imagine a flower in your mind's eye.

Choose any flower you want—a rose, a lily, a tulip—any flower at all as long as it is beautiful.

Now, imagine the flower opening petal by petal, opening, opening, opening until it is fully open.

Add as many details as you want to this visualization, whatever most helps you enjoy it: the shape of the petals, their delicate or bold shading, dewdrops on the flower, a fragrance, perhaps the sound of birdsong in the distance, or sunshine dancing over the flower, coaxing it to open.

Birth Energy

In Creating a Joyful Birth Experience, Capacchione and Bardsley write about connecting with your birth energy, which they describe as a "power from within. . . .which flows through your body, mind, emotions, and spirit. . . .and besides being a natural physical force the *Birth Energy* has an emotional and spiritual dimension, as well."

I like to think of this energy as a reservoir of power and strength, which exists within every woman engaged in the birthing process. It is that part of you that can be called forward to assist, support, and guide you through the birth experience. And as Capacchione and Bardsley indicate, the *Birth Energy* is enriched by the emotional and spiritual bond between mother and baby.

BIRTH ENERGY MEDITATION

The following is a meditation that I have created and shared with pregnant mothers and their partners, which is helpful in accessing the *Birth Energy*

Sit comfortably in your *Sacred Space*. Light a candle. Close your eyes. Breathe in through your nose and then exhale out through your mouth slowly and evenly. Feel the surface that you are resting on, holding and supporting you. Let your body feel that support. Feel the rhythm of your breath breathing through all of your body. Breathing even through your mind. Each breath relaxing you even more deeply. Opening and expanding mind and body. Opening and accessing that part of yourself which contains a reservoir of wisdom, guidance, strength, and support. It is here in this place where your *Birth Energy* resides. In your mind's eye visualize a reservoir that safely holds and honors this powerful dimension of yourself. Perhaps, you will see the *Birth Energy* emerge from the reservoir and/or you may feel the *Birth Energy* energetically in your body.

Allow your breath's rhythm to gently connect to the *Birth Energy*. Feel the two rhythms folding and overlapping into one another; creating one vibrant and dynamic energy together. The *Birth Energy* may feel ever so subtle, or it may crescendo from a faint to a more distinct pulsation. Ride on the waves of whatever you are experiencing. Get a sense of the *Birth Energy's* color, shape, texture, sound, and fragrance. How do you feel in its company? Dialogue with it. Ask it any questions you have, for example . . .Who are you? What are you? What is the best way to call you forth, especially during labor? Is there anything that you need to let me know now? Is there anything that I can do to better prepare for birthing my baby? Will you help my support team? Is there anything you wish to communicate to me from the baby?

When you feel the dialogue is complete, begin to see the *Birth Energy* return to the reservoir within, knowing that you can access it at any time. As you get closer to your due date, you may become more and more aware of this energy's presence— feeling its strength, power, wisdom, and support. For now, bring your attention back to your breath. Breathing in through your nose. Exhaling out slowly and evenly through your mouth. Whenever you are ready, slowly open your eyes.

Write and/or draw in your journal about your experience. If you wish, think of an object that might symbolize this energy. Wear the symbol, put it in your hair, place it on your altar or in some other place where you can be reminded of its presence in your life.

STORIES

No matter how our child might come to us, most parents will agree that destiny or larger unknown forces play a powerful role. Birth stories enchant, inspire, humble, and mystify, while powerfully connecting us to universal feelings of joy, love, pain, and sorrow, and ultimately to each other.

Traditional
- Tibetan women eat lotus buds which have been chanted over by Buddhist monks, so that their body will open up like a lotus flower and give birth easily.
- In some societies, the placenta is cooked and the broth eaten by the mother. Some people plant it in the earth

beneath a young tree, so that the Earth Mother will remain close to the body of that child throughout life.

- There have been accounts of Tlinget women in Alaska giving birth while sleeping!

- The Kwakiutl of British Columbia heat kelp and apply it to the mother's stomach and the small of her back to help ease the pain of labor.

- The Tiwi of Australia press hot leaves against the mother's back, groin, and legs at the beginning of each contraction to help relieve cramping.

- The Aboriginal elder women of Australia cut a piece of the umbilical cord with a stone tool and twist it into a necklace, which the newborn will wear around his or her neck. This is meant to symbolize the baby's connection to the Ancestors.

- The Tibetans in the Himalayas will put saffron powder or yak butter on the tip of the newborn's tongue, so that the baby might speak with wisdom. And before the cord is cut, the father will say a baby blessing, such as, "My child, you have been born from our hearts and souls. May you live one hundred years and see a hundred autumns, may you have a long and glorious life, overcoming all ills and enjoying complete happiness, prosperity, and fortune."

- When the umbilical cord falls off the baby, some Native American tribes slit the bottom of a leather beaded bag (made for this purpose), place the cord inside, and then sew the bag up again. The bag is given to the child's mother to carry with her for the rest of her life. When the mother dies, she is buried with the umbilicus bag, which symbolizes being united forever with her children and Mother Earth.

- Both Cherokee and Tibetans massage their newborns daily to assure proper brain development.

- On the island of Bali, birth is a community event. Babies

are born at home, are most often caught by the father, with the help of the dukun (healer) and a female relative who often supports the woman in a squatting position and massages her abdomen. The female elders of the village provide emotional support while most of the other villagers, including young children, hover nearby. From the moment he takes his first breath, the Balinese child is a child of the whole community, which will support and nurture him throughout his life.

Personal

- Moments after a friend delivered her second daughter in a birthing tub, her four-year-old (who was present for most of the birth) took off all of her clothes, jumped into the water with mommy, daddy, and new baby sister, and exclaimed, "Oh, she's so cute. Let's keep her!"

- On the day a baby girl was born in China, her future mother and father (who had been merely considering adoption at that point) found themselves drawn to an orientation meeting sponsored by an international adoption agency, who would bring baby and parents together nine months later.

- Friends who chose to have their twins delivered by an obstetrician brought their *sacred ground* into the hospital setting. Their *sacred ground* was composed of the items that were used in the *Birth Prayer Ritual:* a silk scarf and Goddess stone carving from their altar, the Native American blanket everyone sat on during the ceremony, the *Baby Bundle,* flowers, and the recorded music played.

- After experiencing a very difficult labor and caesarian birth with her first child, Jane was determined to create a more positive experience with her second. On one cold February morning, Jane went into labor at home. After a very courageous journey, Jane, her partner Ann, their four-year-old daughter Reid, and a midwife joyfully welcomed baby Isabel into the world.

- After many hours of labor, a father whispered to his unborn daughter (at the lower end of the mother's belly), to move from the transverse position that she was in (lying straight across the uterus) into the proper position, so that she could be born without surgery. Shortly after this encouragement, the baby flipped around and was born naturally.

- We gave Zach his first bath when he was several days old. We smudged the space with white sage, lit candles, and to the strains of "Coyote Old Man" (one of the tapes that I listened to when in labor) we tenderly and lovingly bathed our new son in rose water. Zach screamed going in and screamed coming out of the tiny baby tub. But while soaking in the warm rose water, his entire body relaxed. Bathing him in warm water like this and carrying him close to our chests while walking, especially outdoors, seemed to help soothe our newborn during his "colicky" episodes.

The following stories illustrate how family members and friends can share in the birth experience in a sacred and meaningful way.

- On the day Suky's niece was born, she wrote a long letter telling her about the day of her birth. "I included every detail I could remember, beginning with my sighting of a lone juvenile eagle, her c-section arrival, up through the last thing I saw: both parents murmuring to her at one in the morning, exhausted, amazed, and in love."

- My mother presented baby Zach (her seventh grandchild) a scrapbook overflowing with stories and photographs of her own life, beginning when she was a young child, through the time of being a mother and then a grandmother. It also contained photographs and "tales" of my childhood. The gift, honoring grandmother, mother and grandson, sits right next to Zach's baby book.

- Our friend Nelson offered a *Baby Bundle* to Zach when he was one day old. As he presented the beaded infant moccasins, agate coyote fetish, and carnelian stone, Nelson talked about the gift's significance and how each one honored and welcomed Zach's unique song.

- On a warm spring day with cherry blossoms in bloom, we joined friends planting a peach tree in honor of their daughter's birth. For many of us, it was our first opportunity to welcome this new little being into the world. And while gathered around the newly planted tree and the baby girl, who was now cradled in her mother's arms, we offered our prayers and songs.

ADOPTION

Our children seem to come into our lives, as we come into theirs, on some kind of dynamic life-charged energy. This holds true no matter how our child comes to us. I have highlighted the following stories that two families shared with me, which stunningly convey how powerful forces beyond the biological bring family members together.

THE STORY OF EMILY

Wah and his wife May, an elegant couple in their fifties, had been married without children for thirty years. During that time they were self-confessed workaholics, loving their lives and traveling the world. On one of their trips to Hong Kong, they connected with Wah's sister, who was on her way to China to adopt a baby girl. She invited Wah and May to travel with her. They said yes, even though at the time it didn't really seem to make sense. Once in Qing Yuen, Wah and May accompanied Wah's sister to the orphanage. While she was busy doing the required paperwork, Wah and May began to wander the halls. What they saw was heart-wrenching: abandoned babies, ranging from only a few days to three years old—some who had been born in a hospital to mothers who disappeared a few hours later; some who were left in a field or in a train station; others handed over by mothers who themselves had been abandoned by a government that refused them subsidy, or was threatening to take away what they had already been allotted, if they gave birth to a girl.

Eventually, May and Wah found themselves drawn to the crib of a nine-month-old baby girl with "bright eyes and a chubby face." When they each held this little baby in their arms, somehow it just felt right. When Wah went to lay the baby back down, a tear welled up in the child's eyes. Touched by this, Wah picked her up again, and as he brought her to his chest, she grasped his little finger with one of her tiny hands and smiled. Wah melted. He said, "From that moment on, there was no turning back!" Unable to overcome the political and legal obstacles of adopting in that moment, Wah and May were forced to leave China without the baby. After a grueling and anxiety-ridden six months, they were finally granted permission to bring their daughter home.

Wah and May named their daughter Emily, in honor of the great poet, Emily Dickinson, and the prose writer, Emily Bronte. In the first moments of meeting Emily in the orphanage, it seemed clear in their minds they were meant to be a family. Wah and May, like most of us who cross over the threshold into parenthood, say that bringing Emily home changed their lives forever. The presence of Emily, including all of the parent/child challenges and frustrations, has made their lives far richer and more meaningful. And they feel blessed.

The Story of Gabriel

Jeff and Diane knew of Gabe's coming before he was even born across the world in Romania. One warm autumn day Diane, a deeply spiritual woman and gifted psychotherapist, was leading one of her clients in a guided meditation. Midway through the meditation, the client suddenly opened her eyes. She insisted that they stop doing their work together, because she was feeling a "being" in the room—a "Holy Presence" who was bringing a message to Diane. Diane attempted to refocus the session and maintain the professional framework in which she and her client had been working, but her client persisted, eventually relating the following message. "Your soul's longing is about to come true. Your heart's deepest wish has been heard and answered."

Although Diane was puzzled by the relevance of this message to her personally, she could feel the stunning energy and power of something taking place in that moment. The client went on to talk about an extraordinary baby, who would be born in circumstances that were "very poor and decrepit." The final message concluded: "Diane, you and your husband must prepare for what is coming, you and your husband must prepare for this blessing from the angels. It will all unfold in its own time. You have been blessed."

In the preceding months Jeff and Diane, who had a long history of miscarriages, had begun preparations to adopt a child from Romania. In fact, an adoption agency was organizing a trip there for two adoptive families, and Jeff and Diane were hoping to be one of the families going on the next trip.

Three months after Diane's session with her client, Jeff and Diane left for the Midwest to spend the holidays with Diane's family. It was there that they received a phone call from Romania, from the man coordinating the adoptions. With urgency in his voice he said, "There is a baby boy here for you. He was born on December 20. The only problem is that you need to be here in four days!" Miraculously, Jeff and Diane arrived in Romania as quickly as they could, where they were united (or was it reunited?) with their newborn son.

Due to political and legal complications, they were detained for one month, and like Wah and May, they had no idea if they would be able to bring their infant boy home. But despite all of the hardships for both child and parents, the connection remained deep. Jeff believes that it was the "spiritual bonding" that helped them overcome these difficulties. He also feels strongly that the spiritual bond is what has helped heal some of the physical and emotional wounds that Gabriel endured in the earliest days of his life.

Shortly after returning home together, Jeff and Diane had a baby-naming ceremony. Even before they had arrived in Romania, they knew that Gabriel would be the name of their son. "It was as though his name had been chosen for him." Now they wanted to celebrate his arrival with close friends and family. In their gathering circle, a rabbi talked about how Jeff, Diane, and Gabriel had come together. Jeff himself shared, "Gabe came to earth and called us to come and get him. He magnetically held out his hand across the ocean and reached out to us. We reached back with our hands, and in that instant, we became a family."

RITUALS, CEREMONIES, AND CELEBRATIONS

Baby Bundle, Baby-Naming Ceremony, and *Planting A Tree* are lovely ways that you, your family, and friends can welcome and celebrate your newborn's arrival. *Welcoming the Soul of a Child Healing Ritual* offers a sacred way in which you can celebrate your baby's birth, while acknowledging his soul's song. It is a ritual that also can be used to heal any difficulties or trauma that may have arisen during labor and birth.

Baby Bundle

A *Baby Bundle* is a gift containing meaningful symbols and prayers for the newborn child. It can be presented at many of the rituals and ceremonies honoring the birth. You can create the gift alone, with your birth partner, your children, or at a gathering with your loved ones. Whatever you decide, creating the *Baby Bundle* can be a wonderful welcoming ritual for your baby.

Days or weeks before the actual ceremony, you might begin to gather or make meaningful items to be placed into the *Baby Bundle*. Allow your inner wisdom, the baby, your ancestors, and the Divine to guide you. Bring those items to the ceremony where you actually will make the *Baby Bundle*.

In your *sacred space* lay out all of your materials that will be used: perhaps a piece of fabric to serve as the outer wrapping of the bundle and whatever you will use to decorate the outer wrapping (paints, pens, embroidery thread, feathers, beads, stones, etc.). Also bring the gifts that you have already gathered to place inside of the bundle. The inside gifts are best kept simple and symbolic (a colored candle, a prayer bead, a tiny felt doll, a stone, or fetish). Before creating and assembling the *Baby Bundle* light a candle, burn white sage (to purify the space and materials), and then bless the materials and gifts. Put on some favorite music and create!

Once the *Baby Bundle* is made, consider it a sacred object that can be used in any of the rituals, placed on your altar or in your baby's room or make it part of the *sacred ground* created for labor and birth. You can also present the *Baby Bundle* to your child at any time as a way to welcome and honor his birth.

Baby-Naming Ceremony

Humans are a chant singing their song to God. Every time the name is spoken, the name vibrates an

energy. Each vibration is connected to another . . .
when the name is spoken, healing happens.

BEAUTIFUL PAINTED ARROW

Gather together with loved ones in a garden, a park, on someone's front porch, in the room where your child was conceived or where he was born (if at home). Have everyone sit in a circle. Make an altar in the center of the ceremonial space with candles, flowers, gifts for the baby, etc. Wrap the baby in his receiving blanket. Hold the baby or lay him down on soft blankets near you. Say a prayer or share words that express the purpose of his ritual. Talk about how you have come to choose the name of this child, and the name's significance. Pass around a basket of small tapered candles so that each person can take one. You and your birth partner light your candles first, and then with your candles light a special one for your new child. As you light his candle, you can offer a prayer, a blessing, a chant, or a song. If you have other children, have them light their candle from yours next. Then pass the light on to each person until everyone's candle is lit. Invite those gathered to share a blessing or story, if they wish to. Close the ritual with a chant, song, poem, or reading. Celebrate by sharing food and drink, music and dancing!

Planting a Tree

Planting a tree to honor the birth of a child is a practice that dates back to ancient times. In some traditions it represents a long, healthy, and happy life. To others it symbolizes rooting ourselves in the earth as we unfold and blossom into our fullest beauty and potential. A certain type of tree might symbolize the qualities that are meant to be awakened within a child during his life. Ted Andrews offers a section on the symbolic qualities of trees and flowers in his fascinating book, *Animal-Speak: The Spiritual and Magical Powers of Creatures Great and Small.* Apple symbolizes beauty and happiness; lilac, the realization of one's true beauty, walnut, following a unique path. All in all, it is a ravishing way to mark the birth and life of a new child.

To select a tree, pay attention to what trees come to you in dreams or which ones you naturally gravitate to. You can also ask your newborn (via a nondominant handwriting exercise, dialoguing, or a visualization) to give an opinion. Always trust your intuition. Whatever you choose will be perfect.

Select and prepare the planting site. (You might choose a site first, and consider what types of trees grow best there). It might be in your backyard, on a friend's piece of property, in a park, or even in a clay pot.

Invite family and friends. Gather in a circle around the planting site. Open with a prayer, blessing, or reading. Share, in your own words, the purpose of this ceremony. Talk about the symbolism of the tree. As part of the ritual you can have everyone help dig into the earth and prepare the soil for planting, or do this ahead of time. Plant, pat down the soil, and water the tree together. (Little ones particularly like to be helpful, and it is a wonderful opportunity for them to feel involved and connected to the newest member of the family/community.) Bring the circle closer around the tree, hold hands and share prayer offerings and stories, or simply stand in silence. Bless the tree. Bless the child.

Celebrate with a picnic, indoors or outdoors. Play music and dance around the tree.

Welcoming the Soul of a Child Celebration

This ritual can be a beautiful and joyful welcoming celebration or can be adapted as a healing ceremony for a birth experience that may have been extremely difficult. With a new appreciation for the tremendous impact that the birth experience has on the development of our children, I recently designed this ritual for my husband, son, and myself. Having the experience together was poignant and deeply healing.

Before performing this ritual, reread the story of the African tribe as told on the first page in this book's Introduction. Our son was five when we did this ceremony together, so we told him the story first. This gave him an opportunity to ask questions and to share his own thoughts about the custom and what he thought the soul was. Since Zach loves to "act," presenting the ritual as a story engaged him from the very beginning.

You will need: A tree or something that symbolizes a tree, sage or incense, candles, matches, flowers, cushions or a blanket to sit on, a symbol of the birth, a piece of fabric to wrap the symbol in during the ritual, a basket of small white candles, and a gift for the child.

Select a sacred place, indoors or outdoors. Create a ceremonial circle with stones, cushions, or a blanket. Make an altar in the middle of the circle, which can include flowers, candles, and any sacred earth objects. If you are doing the ritual outdoors, create the circle near a beautiful tree; if you are indoors use a potted tree or something that can symbolize a tree.

Begin the ritual by having your guests take a seat around the sacred circle. Then mother, father, and baby or child (whose birth is being healed and celebrated) come into the middle of the circle together. Purify the space with sage or incense. Light a candle. State the purpose of this ritual and, if you wish, say a prayer or blessing. If the purpose is to heal a difficult or traumatic birth, state that in your opening prayers. Bring into the circle a symbol of the birth. Share your feelings and thoughts about the birth. What did this experience teach or heal? If the ritual is serving as a healing experience, after sharing your thoughts and feelings about the birth, wrap the symbol up in a piece of fabric. Either bury it under leaves or in the ground, or burn it. You can do this as part of the ritual now or later.

If the ceremony is purely for celebration, place the symbol in the middle of the circle along with the other sacred objects.

Now you are going to re-enact *listening* for your child's song. Either have someone narrate the story as you go along, or read it aloud before this part of the ritual begins. The mother leaves the circle and goes to the tree. There *"she sits and listens for the song"* of her unborn child. Bring the baby near the tree in a blanket. If needed, have a loved one hold him.

If your child is older, have him quietly leave the circle and sit near the tree as his mother *listens* quietly. When he is ready to express his song, he can sing, hum, move/dance around his mother, recite a poem, or simply say, "Here I am. I'm ready to be born." You can talk about this beforehand, or you may allow for pure spontaneity. Who knows? Maybe you will see your child's soul emanating through!

Once hearing the *song,* the mother returns to the circle and teaches it to her partner. (The baby or child can return with the mother to the circle as well, or, if older, the child may want to sit or move around the circle's outer rim.) Mother and father now sing the *song* together as they hold each other lovingly, then teach the *song* to the "midwives and elders" (your loved ones); they can now join in as well and sing the *song* with you. Or you might invite everyone to play a percussion instrument or chant together, "We welcome you (child's name). We welcome you."

The mother now reenacts the birth with the support of loved ones. Using human bodies, cushions, a nylon retractable tunnel or tent, create a birth canal for the child to go through; this can be deeply healing, as it can offer a more gentle, loving, and caring birth experience. When the baby is "born," everyone welcomes him with oohs and aahs, hugs and kisses (only if the child or baby is comfortable with this). The *song* is then sung again together.

If you wish, share your feelings, along with your partner and child. Your loved ones may wish to do so as well. Pass around a basket with small tapered candles. Mother or father light the first candle, saying something like, "May each candle that is lighted illuminate our life's path . . . always bringing light and lightness . . . as we travel, sometimes together, sometimes apart . . . May each candle express our growing and expanding love for this child . . . We welcome you (child's name) and feel so blessed that you have come." As everyone lights a candle, they can say also prayers or share whatever they feel like saying. Or you might choose to do this part of the ritual in complete silence first. Simply watching the light become brighter and brighter as each candle is lit can be a very moving experience. Once all of the candles are lit, join with your loved ones in the outer circle. Place your baby in the inner circle, or guide your older child there. For a moment or two (or however long it is possible) surround this child, lovingly, with lighted candles and open hearts. If you wish, present a gift. (At a summer Wilderness Awareness camp, Zach was given the fox as an animal totem. So, in this ceremony we gave him a hand-carved fox fetish made from alabaster). Close the ritual by giving thanks and gratitude. Sing the child's *song* again, read from something that you have composed or chosen for this occasion, or get up and dance. Celebrate and let your child know how loved and welcome he is in your world.

5

Living Together Amongst the Sacred Trees
UNFOLDING AND BLOSSOMING

Once when Zach was three, he woke up in the middle of the night. He said that he couldn't sleep and wanted me to hold him. As he lay in my arms, I could feel that he was slightly warm, and figured that he wasn't feeling well. After getting him a sip of water and walking with him, we ended up on our study's wine-colored sofa. I stretched out on my back with Zach resting on top of my chest. As we lay there quietly, the moon reflected its light upon the snowy fields outside our window, lavishing us in its glow. I remember how struck I was by the stillness; the only sound, the gentle in and out of Zach's breath. Just as he surrendered back into sleep, I experienced the most stunning thing. With his head curled up in my neck and his heart directly over mine, I could feel how different Zach's heart felt from my own. My heart felt like a tightly closed rose, with its petals intricately wrapped and folded inward. It was a bloom that had somehow forgotten to reopen itself in the early morning sunlight. Zach's heart, in contrast, felt like an immense field of high meadow wildflowers, vibrantly colored, fragrant, and pulsating full of life. I closed my eyes. I let myself enter into the moment with this tiny creature, a little dalai lama, who had come into my world to teach me to love again.

"Do not be afraid to love," says poet and Zen Master Thich Nhat Hanh. "Without love, life is impossible . . . without love, a child cannot flower, an adult cannot mature. Without love, we weaken, wither."

Our children have come to our world to teach us how to love again. If we are paying attention, we can see how they invite us, in every moment, to deepen, grow, and open. In fact, they give us the opportunity (often, without choice!) to cultivate all of the great skills integral to a spiritual practice, such as loving kindness, mindfulness, compassion, and forgiveness.

In many indigenous societies, the community sees children as perfect teachers who come through the bodies of their parents, but belong to the whole community. This view is intrinsic to cultures that believe everyone comes to this life with a purpose. Therefore, it is the responsibility of the people in that community to nurture, respect, and honor each child—to be the safe-keepers of their soul's journey.

Most of us, however, feel alienated from our community and from our family and friends, rather than honored. We need to find ways to reconnect with one another—to heal and transform our wounds rather than to use them as a shield to hide behind and distance ourselves from ourselves and each other. When we become solely identified with our wounds and a story, we virtually forget who we truly are. If we are stuck in replaying past events, it is impossible to be in the present, "the only place where love is found," and truly connect with our lives and each other. To honor our wound is to enter into the heart of the pain and to allow the pain to lead us to the deepest expression of our self, back into our own true hearts where the gifts and treasures of our soul awaits us.

"We have to learn the art of loving. We need to support each other to build communities where love is tangible. When we touch the present moment deeply, we also touch the past . . . we have to let the ancestors in us be liberated. The moment that we can offer them joy, peace, and freedom, we offer joy, peace, and freedom to ourselves, our children, and their children at the same time." (Thich Nhat Hanh)

Babies and children just by their presence alone can help us transform our world, for they are our ambassadors for humanity; teaching and inspiring us to crack open the encrusted mantle that encases our hearts.

> *I want to unfold*
> *Let no place in me hold itself closed*
> *for where I am closed, I am false.*
> *I want to stay clear in your sight . . .*
> *I want to free what waits within me.*
> —RAINER MARIA RILKE

RAPHAELA

Maria, a lovely friend who has always been devoted to her spiritual path, was ecstatic when she learned of her pregnancy, for she and her husband, Jonathan, had dreamed about having a child together for some time. Around the beginning of her second trimester, Maria was astounded when she began to experience feelings of intense anger. These feelings eventually manifested into uncomfortable chest pains. Investigating the pain enabled Maria to get in touch with the tremendous anger that she still carried in response to her mother's inability to love. Concerned that her baby would be born into this energy of anger, Maria went deeper into her work around this issue with her mother.

Around this time, Maria took a workshop with the well-known energy healer, Rosylyn Bruyere. Early on in the workshop, Rosylyn invited Maria to lie down in the center of the room, and asked all of the workshop participants to gather around her. There, with Rosylyn's hands placed on Maria's chest, the group became a safe, nourishing, and loving womb, tenderly holding Maria and her unborn baby. Within moments, Maria's chest pains went away. This striking experience gave to her what she describes as "a model of the village and how we don't have to be alone in our pain." Inspired by her love for her unborn daughter, Raphaela, Maria courageously journeyed into the depths of her pain, to heal a wound endured when she was very small. And Raphaela, a teacher and healer at four months in utero, was already singing her soul's song.

PARENTING AS A SPIRITUAL PATH.

A friend who had the privilege of meeting Mother Theresa asked how she might create a more spiritual and meaningful life. Mother Theresa asked her if she had children, to which the answer was yes. She then said, "Go home, be with your children, and love them with all of your heart. This is your spiritual practice."

Hindus teach that there are two paths to spiritual initiation: one is through living in a monastery, and the other through parenting. In Tibet, caring for the children is a sacred practice of the entire community. A similar belief is held by many tribes of Africa. For many indigenous cultures, seeing the sacred in children, and in all of life, is so intrinsic to who they are that they don't delineate or separate the spiritual from any part of their day-to-day living.

Parenting as a Spiritual Path is about waking up and being as conscious as we possibly can in our relationship to ourselves, our children, and to our world, to honor the interconnectedness of all of life. Parenting with this intention takes courage, commitment, devotion, and love in its purest sense. Conscious or mindful parenting is an arduous spiritual discipline, one that illuminates our innate goodness and our capacity to love, while in the same breath, revealing the most hidden, disowned, and unloved aspects of our self. The moment that we "call forth" our children into our life, they beckon us to be dedicated to our own healing journey.

Myla and Jon Kabat-Zinn clearly capture the challenge of parenting in their inspiring book, *Everyday Blessings: The Inner Work of Mindful Parenting*. "As with any spiritual discipline, the call to parent mindfully is filled with enormous promise and potential. Parenting mindfully also challenges us to do the inner work on ourselves to be fully adequate to the task, so that we can be fully engaged in this hero's journey, this quest of a lifetime that is a human life lived . . . the very fact that we are a parent is continually asking us to find and express what is most nourishing, most loving, most wise and caring in ourselves, to be, as much as we can, our best selves."

Parenting as a path offers a framework for being in our life with our children in a more conscious and meaningful way; a touchstone for keeping us on course. When approaching parenthood as a path, we are presented with the profoundest of teaching opportunities—daily. It's no great wonder why, in the spirit of fun, yet with humbling accuracy, we refer to our children as Zen masters, lamas, little Buddhas, and gurus. The truth of their teaching ranks with the holiest of holies—and we don't even need to cross the widest oceans or ascend the steepest peaks to be in their presence. But our children will dare us to travel to places we thought unimaginable. As we journey through the ever-changing landscape of parenthood, we will experience profound awe, wonder, and joy. We will also feel unprepared, scared, confused, and lost.

The Kabat-Zinns eloquently talk about how mindful parenting is best seen as a *practice,* a discipline. *Practice* means "embodying wholeness right now . . . intentionally remembering to be fully present with whatever comes up, so that you are not always on automatic pilot or acting mechanically. When you are picking up the baby, you are there with picking up the baby. When you are hugging your child, you are there with hugging your child . . . Every moment is our teacher. Each child, each circumstance, each breath is our teacher. It is all here, waiting to be embraced right now, in this moment."

Parenting as a spiritual path is exquisitely personal and individual. There are infinite opportunities to deepen our spiritual practice, yet unfortunately there is little support in our culture to honor parenting in this way. Sadly, this has created a huge void in our society. If the notion of parenting as a spiritual path invokes something deep within you, your practice has already begun. Go deeper by exploring your own spiritual beliefs and practices. How might these beliefs and practices embrace parenting as part of your teaching? Or how might parenting enhance, strengthen, challenge, deepen, and embrace your spiritual seeking? Dialogue with your partner, friends, and family about how you might integrate spirituality into your home and into your community of families. Plan informal gatherings, share food, conversation, moments of silence, laughter, and tears. Listen to your souls singing.

Recently I met Jon, who with his wife Betsy, is exploring parenting as a spiritual path with six other couples. They have met every other Sunday for the past year with Mary Grace Lentz, a facilitator of parenting groups, practicing Buddhist, and mother of two. Although everyone in the group comes from diverse religious backgrounds and beliefs, their passionate commitment to parenting their children consciously links them together. They begin each session with five or ten minutes of silence for the purpose of practicing being fully present. (The children, ages several months to eleven years old, are integral to these gatherings and take turns ringing the meditation bell). And although a parent may need to tend to his or her child, everyone practices sitting together quietly. After this, the group will usually share something about how their spiritual practice is going or they may discuss "homework" that was assigned in their last session. As a group they then may explore a topic, or talk about a book that the group is reading (such as *Everyday*

Blessings). Sometimes they go on a family retreat, share dinner, or take a walk, but they always do so in the spirit of including and honoring the children. Through intention, dialoguing, practice, and supporting one another, these parents are hoping to permeate their homes with harmony, clarity, and compassion. They provide wonderful inspiration and a model on how to strengthen, deepen, and support our spiritual path through parenting.

Jack Kornfield says, "Parenting is a labor of love. It's a path of service and surrender and, like the practice of a Buddha or bodhisattva (a seeker of enlightenment), it demands patience, understanding, and tremendous sacrifice. It is also a way to reconnect with the mystery of life."

Parenting as a Spiritual Path asks us to be present, authentic, and more vibrantly alive. If we are more conscious and awake we are then able to see our children, and ourselves for that matter, without the dense protective lens that tints the truth and magnificence of any moment.

Throughout this book, *Cultivating Skills, Exercises, Rituals, Ceremonies and Celebrations* are intended to enrich your spiritual path, while fostering a deeper sense of presence and connection to your life. Integrating *Parenting as a Spiritual Path* naturally begins to instill extraordinary qualities of connection: to the universal unity of all living things, to our God, to our life's purpose, and to those we love, most especially our children.

CULTIVATING SKILLS

Loving Kindness, Creating a Spiritual Practice with Our Children, Family Traditions, Celebrations and Rituals and *Welcoming the Soul of the Family* can be challenging yet invaluable disciplines and practices that deepen and enrich our connection to our spirituality and to the song of our souls.

Loving Kindness

The practice of *loving kindness,* inspired by the teachings of Buddha, is what some refer to as "the path of heart," a path that acknowledges and embraces the intrinsic goodness of oneself and of others. It can be a rigorous practice, but one that greatly benefits ourselves, others, and especially our children. For it is a practice of opening our heart, which "uncovers the radiant, joyful heart within each of us and manifests this radiance to the world. . . . We find, beneath the wounding concepts of separation, a connection both to ourselves and to all beings." *(Lovingkindness* by Sharon Salzberg).

The value of cultivating this skill in relationship to parenting our children is that, in coming from *loving kindness,* we naturally remedy many of the unfulfilled needs and desires that were most likely passed down to us, from our family and culture, and then on to our own children. Through a *loving kindness* practice we are less likely to project onto our children our own unresolved and frustrating feelings of unworthiness, unhappiness, or unloveableness, and are therefore better able to honor and appreciate our children for who they really are in the most genuine sense. When we break from the unconscious patterns, we give our children a healthier environment in which they can flourish.

Ultimately, through our healing work and with a dedicated *loving kindness* practice (see *Lovingkindness Meditation),* we open our heart to ourselves, to others, and most importantly to our children, whom we will encourage to blossom into their most radiant beauty as they sing their soul's song.

Creating a Spritual Practice with Our Children

Young children are naturally connected to their spirit. We were, too, when we were little. The yearning that I hear adults talk about in my work is often the longing for reconnection to that which we, as individuals and as a culture, have become so alienated from: our spirit and soul. Our children can help us rediscover our innate connection to the parts of ourselves that we have lost and to a more meaningful life, for they embody spirit. They are curious, imaginative, creative, adventurous, genuine, delighted by the ordinary, are playful and loving, in awe of the natural world, and totally in the moment.

To create a spiritual practice with your children, first connect with what "arouses your spirit." Think of what inspires you. What makes you feel deeply connected to your life, to your loved ones, to all living things? What helps you experience your life in a meaningful way? What makes your heart open? What makes you experience joy? If your children are old enough, ask them to think about these things, too. Contemplating these questions will begin to guide you to where you naturally and authentically express your own spirituality.

For many of us, we have already created the elements of a spiritual practice, but probably haven't identified it as such. It may be simply bringing more attention and intention to what we already are doing. A good example is adding to or enhancing something you and your child do every day together. Create a good morning blessing song and sing it together as you pull open the curtains in their bedroom, or while they are getting dressed. Express thanks for the food you are preparing and eating. Invite a child to sit on your lap when you meditate or read inspiring words. Have them stretch with you when you are doing yoga or a deep-breathing exercise. Take a walk together and have them listen to the language of the birds, or watch the sunrise or sunset. As part of your bedtime ritual, include a special poem, quote, prayer, meditation, or tell a story which expresses compassion and kindness. Tell your child what you appreciate about her. Say a blessing when you turn off the lights, or when you switch on the night light. If you aren't sure where to begin, simply go into the stillness and ask

how you might share spirituality in your life. Ask your child in *Communing with the Soul of a Child Meditation.*

A lovely gift is given to your child every time she sees you expressing your spirituality. In this context, I am not really talking about religion, which I see as a formalized practice based on doctrine and tradition—although your spirituality may be expressed in your religious practice. Expressing your spirituality is intimately personal. It is when you see glimpses of your soul coming through, and where your heart and soul sings. It is the experience of feeling your oneness with all of life. You may connect with your spirituality while praying, when expressing gratitude while sitting in a garden, before sharing a meal with dear friends, or with your child before he/she falls asleep. Or you may connect to your spirituality through your love for storytelling, music, art, drumming, dancing, chanting, meditating, reading, writing, being with friends, gardening, caring for animals, cooking, playing, walking on a beach or beneath a canopy of cedars, giving service, creating a ritual, or simply enjoying a moment of quiet. One of the fondest memories that I have with my grandfather was joining him for his walk at the end of the day, up to the top of a hilly street where we would watch the sunset in complete silence. Although I was probably only six or seven, I vividly remember feeling a sense of oneness with the golden colors in the sky and with the man who was tenderly holding my hand.

NATURE AS A TEACHER

It is in nature where I have always felt the deepest connection to my spirituality. It is where I experience being touched by the Divine. So as soon as I could start carrying Zach in a baby backpack, I'd bundle him up and set off for a walk into the lovely ancient hills that cradled our farmhouse in upstate New York. Sometimes I'd sing to Zach his favorite silly songs, point out coyote tracks or whisper to him when we'd come across a herd of white-tailed deer. But the magic for me was listening to the song of the woods: the wind whirling through the white birch and elm, icy cold springwater finding its way down the hillside, and the sustained calling whistle of a red-tailed hawk, a wondrous and exquisite accompaniment to Zach's own sweet sighs, coos, and gurgles. I was in heaven.

He must have been, too. Often the fresh air, sounds, and rhythm of my walking would lull Zach into a restful sleep. I remember the first time I didn't hear or feel any life coming from the papoose on my back, I panicked. It was only after pulling the pack off my back and seeing him, not only sleeping, but wearing a smile of bliss on his face, that I realized that my trekking partner enjoyed these outings as much as I did. At six, he still delights in taking walks, although I can assure you that they include countless side trips, detours, and rest stops. Zach has become a great reminder to slow down and marvel at each wondrous thing that we meet along the path. We particularly like to give special attention to the animals that we come across, for we believe—as do many of the cultures that live close to the earth—that animals are spirit messengers carrying sacred teachings. I have found these moments of sharing to be wonderful ways to feel connected to Zach and to the wisdom of the natural world.

Jon Young, founder and director of The Wilderness Awareness School, uses nature or "coyote teaching" as a way to help individuals reconnect with their spirit. The school is designed for people of all ages, and not surprisingly, Jon says that children need less direction because they are already so connected to the present and to their spirit. "Just watch how they engage all of their senses, their imagination, creativity, and heart when they are outside," he observes. Tragically, "Our society erodes this natural connection over time." As parents and as a world, it is essential to help our children preserve their natural desire and ability to experience and express their spirit. As adults, we need to heal what Jon calls the "cysts of grief" or childhood memories, which along with our cultural trends, result in our break with our spirit. Jon refers to his teaching as "The Art Of Mentoring," which is "a collection of teachings from around the world that examines the universal growth needs of the human spirit and mind, with respect to our relationship to nature and to other human beings and to our own creativity." The Wilderness Awareness School provides a powerful way to help parents and their children strengthen and deepen their connection to their spirit, to each other, and to the great teachings of the natural world; elements integral to any spiritual practice. (See *Resource Guide* to learn more about Jon Young and The Wilderness Awareness School programs, which are offered throughout the country).

When teaching, Jon Young encourages his students to find a "secret spot" outside, near their home, where they are to sit every day for at least five minutes. If you can sit there longer, all the better, as it usually takes about twenty minutes for the disturbance that you just created (by coming into this place) to quiet down, and for nature to return to its own rhythms and sounds. I've been told that if you go to your "secret spot" for the sunrise, as the sunlight travels across the earth from east to west, you can literally hear the birds awakening along the same path. If you are present with all of your senses, you will literally hear and feel their morning song roll right over you and your "secret spot." "The Dawn's Chorus"—a wave of singing, delicately yet powerfully stirring awake our own true heart.

The natural world is a sacred temple where great spiritual teachings can be remembered, cultivated, practiced, and shared. Whether you live in a rural or urban setting, you can bring the teaching into your home. Even if you are an inner city dweller, you can plant seedlings in little pots for a windowsill, or have your child sit on your lap, look out the window, and create a sky, a tree, or a bird meditation. Put up a wind chime or a bird feeder. Make a doorway blessing (a decorative piece to hang over your door), or a centerpiece for your kitchen table, made from flowers, branches, leaves, berries, and herbs, which you can gather on a walk outdoors. Select a tree in your yard or in a park and think of it as what Denise Linn calls in her book, *Sacred Space,* a Guardian Tree. Think of the tree as a source of nourishment and healing for your home and family. Many tribal people believe that trees have souls. Sit or stand next to your chosen tree regularly. Feel its energy supporting you. Ask its spirit or soul to permeate your home with its strength, resiliency, and beauty. Wherever you go, imagine the Guardian Tree's healing energy with you. When we lived in rural New York, our Guardian Tree was an ancient sycamore that stood in the middle of a fallow field. We loved to stand next to its magnificent body, which seemed to hold the wisdom of the ages. Once we found a smooth sculpted branch that had fallen on the ground. After asking the tree permission to take it home, we stretched our connected hands around its immense and pulsating body and gave it thanks. Be certain to always give the tree thanks for sharing its power with you and your family. Some Native Americans call this act "gifting," giving something in return for a gift received in nature. You can express your thanks with a mental thank you, an actual gift (a flower, a crystal, or colorful stone—something natural) or your time (caring for the tree and its environment, picking up litter). Gifting is a simple but powerful practice that awakens a respect and gratitude for all of life.

In their rich book *Celebrating the Great Mother,* Cait Johnson and Maura D. Shaw offer practical and easy-to-follow activities to help families reclaim their spiritual roots through nature. They believe that "by giving children a direct and joyous experience of their connection with the earth, with other people, and the divine, we give them the key not only to personal soul. Another family doesn't believe that there is a language or one word to describe their family's soul, but when they sleep out underneath the stars together, they experience their collective soul being nourished.

Communing with the Soul of the Family Meditation and *Welcoming the Family Soul Ritual* may provide meaningful ways to illuminate, honor, give voice to, and express the family soul and/or the family soul's purpose.

Family Traditions, Celebrations, and Rituals

Creating family traditions, celebrations, and rituals that are personal and meaningful enhances and strengthens our connection to all of our life. Children love celebrations and rituals, because they provide the *sacred ground* from which they can begin to explore and access their own inner wisdom and potential, while feeling safe and connected to themselves and to the family. A family that has traditions and rituals naturally fosters closeness, trust, safety, and a strong sense of connection; qualities that are particularly helpful when we are facing any of life's challenges.

Creating and practicing family traditions, celebrations, and rituals is the family's soul expressing itself. What do yours reflect about your family soul? Think about what you already do as a family that, with just a little more awareness and purpose, might deepen your connection to one another and foster more appreciation. Most often, it is the seemingly ordinary things we do that become our sacred traditions, celebrations, and rituals. Bathe your child with a song or a blessing, take a moment together and watch the colors change in the sky at sunset, light a candle at the dinner table while reciting a prayer or poem and tell your child what you appreciate about her before saying good night. See *Family Traditions, Celebrations, and Rituals Exercise* for other suggestions.

wholeness and health, but to the health of the planet
they will one day inherit."

The great naturalist John Muir said, "Every natural
is a conductor of divinity." Find ways to acknowledge, I
and celebrate your connection to the wisdom of the r
world. Allow your spirit and soul to awaken. (See *R
mended Reading* for other resources on nature as a tea

There are infinite ways in which to express your spiri
and to remember your interconnectedness to all of life.
creating a spiritual practice with your children, the im|
thing is to make it a positive and meaningful experie
them. You will need to be patient, flexible, and open. '
a regular practice. But always follow your children's le
listen to their cues. It is there you will see them expressii
own spirit—opening and blossoming petal by petal in
most authentic and truest selves.

Welcoming the Soul of the Family

When we come together and create a family, no ma
configuration of that family, we birth a spirit and soul
we need to welcome and honor the soul of our child,
to acknowledge the family soul. A favorite family trac
ritual, a symbol, a piece of art, a special room, a word (
a favorite song, musician, movie, place, book, play, a
type of food, what makes you laugh or cry together,
provide important clues and insights into what migł
the essence of your family's soul. If you connect with
the important thing is to acknowledge and honor it.
symbol, a song, ritual, or ceremony to integrate it i
minds, bodies, and hearts. One family has photogra
books about orca whales on their family altar. For the
whales embody beauty, grace, and a powerful link to
dom of their ancestry; qualities they feel reflect their

EXERCISES

When we come together and create a family, we birth a family soul. The following exercises help to acknowledge and honor the soul of the family and develop ways to express our spirituality, in addition to communing with and honoring the soul of our child.

Loving Kindness

This meditation can be found in *Buddha's Little Instruction Book* by Jack Kornfield. It has been especially helpful whenever I am going through a difficult time—be it with myself, a situation, or another person. In addition to reflecting on the phrase given in Kornfield's meditation while meditating, I have also used the phrase when walking in the woods, driving my car, before falling asleep at night, and (my favorite time) when floating on my back, after swimming laps. May it be useful to you in cultivating a happy and open heart.

LOVING KINDNESS MEDITATION

With a loving heart as the background, all that we attempt, all that we encounter will open and flow more easily. Loving kindness meditation uses phrases, images, and feelings to evoke a loving kindness and friendliness toward oneself and others. It is best to practice this meditation for fifteen or twenty minutes daily in a quiet place.

Sit in a comfortable fashion. Let your body rest and be relaxed. Let your heart be soft, letting go of plans and preoccupations. Then begin to recite inwardly the following phrase directed to yourself. You begin with yourself because without loving yourself it is almost impossible to love others.

> May I be filled with loving kindness.
> May I be well.

May I be peaceful and at ease.
May I be happy.

As you repeat these phrases, you can picture yourself as a young and beloved child, or sense yourself as you are now, held in a heart of loving kindness. Adjust the words and images in any way you need to find the exact phrases that best open your heart of kindness. Repeat the phrases over and over again, letting the feelings permeate your body and mind. Practice this meditation for a number of weeks, until the sense of loving kindness for yourself grows.

Be aware that this meditation may at times feel mechanical or awkward, or even bring up feelings contrary to loving kindness, feelings of irritation and anger. If this happens, it is especially important to be patient and kind toward yourself, allowing whatever arises to be received in a spirit of friendliness and kind affection.

When you feel you have established some sense of loving kindness, you can then expand your meditation to include others in the same meditation period. After first focusing on yourself, choose someone in your life who has truly cared for you. Picture this person and carefully recite the same phrases: *May he/may she be filled with loving kindness,* and so forth. When loving kindness for this person has developed, begin to include other people you love in the meditation, picturing each one and reciting the same phrases, evoking a sense of loving kindness for them.

After this you can include others: friends, community members, neighbors, people everywhere, animals, all beings, the whole earth. Include the difficult people in your life, wishing that they, too, be filled with loving kindness and peace. In the course of twenty minutes your meditation can open from yourself to loved ones, to all beings everywhere.

Loving kindness can be practiced anywhere. You can use this meditation in traffic jams, in buses and airplanes. As you silently practice this meditation among people, you will imme-diately feel a wonderful connection with them—the power of loving kindness. It will calm your life and keep you connected to your heart.

Communing with the Soul of Your Child Meditation

This guided meditation provides a wonderful opportunity to connect to the spirit or soul of your child. I may do this in one of my regular meditation sessions or I may do it right after Zach has fallen asleep. I especially like to do it right after he falls asleep, because I can feel his energy still electrifying the room. I might sit on his bed or on the floor next to his bed and then guide myself though the experience. The meditation may last anywhere from a few moments to fifteen or twenty minutes. Leave your child in the meditation with loving thoughts.

Regarding this meditation, some of my clients have asked how you distinguish your own "inner child" (an aspect of our personality which often expresses feelings, emotions, and beliefs of our child-self) from the spirit or soul of your "in-the-flesh" child. If you are unsure, simply ask the child when he or she appears in the meditation, "Are you the voice or image of my inner child, or are you the voice of (your child's name)?"

Sit comfortably. Bring your attention to your breath, breath-ing in fully through your nose, breathing gently and evenly out through the mouth. Breathing in. Breathing out. Allow your breath to do what it knows to do. In and out. So effortless and easy. Breathing in and breathing out. Each breath carrying you into a deep place of ease. Feel the surface beneath you completely holding and supporting you.

When you feel ready, imagine a special place where you would like to be with your child. It may be a place that you and your child have been to together, or it may be somewhere new. In either case, it should be a sacred place where you can come together, safely and comfortably. Imagine yourself there now. Allow all of your senses to experience this place fully. Then, whenever you are ready, invite your child to join you. Allow your child to come in her own time and in her own way. You may see or sense her at the age that she is now currently, or you may see her as younger or older. She may even appear as an animal or as a symbol. When you feel ready, ask a question, such as "Is there anything that you wish to tell me? Is there anything that I need to know? Is there anything that I can do now to help you on your life's journey?" Now *listen* . . . Your child may speak to you in words, show you what she feels or needs, or bring you a symbolic gift. You may end up having a dialogue, or you may find yourself just "hanging out" together.

When your time together feels complete, tell your child that you can come together in this way anytime. Thank her for meeting you here and sharing whatever she shared with you. Express your deepest love to her. Then return your attention to your breath, breathing in through your nose fully, breathing out through the mouth slowly and evenly. Feel the surface beneath you, holding and supporting you. Whenever you are ready, slowly open your eyes.

Communing with the Soul of the Family Meditation

This guided meditation is a variation of *Communing with the Soul of Your Child Meditation*. Follow the same outline, but when you come to inviting your child to your special place, invite the soul of your family. The soul of the family may appear consistently as a specific symbol, or it may present itself in a myriad of ways at different times. You may connect to something visually, or you may get an overall "felt sense" of the soul. You might ask the soul questions such as, "What is it that you wish to communicate to me in this moment? How is it that we have come together in this lifetime? What is our family soul's purpose? What can we do individually and/or as a family to help our family soul to grow, strengthen, heal, or evolve? What is the family soul's song?"

Practice the meditation separately or do it with your partner or even with the entire family (see *Welcoming the Family Soul Ritual*). Afterwards, share your experiences. Write in your journals. Talk about what you have learned. How might you put into action any insights gained? What do you think your family's soul song is? You can always benefit from doing this meditation when a family member or the entire family is facing a challenge. Or better yet, do it as a scheduled family ritual once a week or once a month.

The Family Talking Stick

In the Native American culture, the Talking Stick is a branch or twig from a tree, blessed and adorned with meaningful objects, such as feathers, beads, and fetishes, that is used in council meetings to assure that each and every person is heard with respect and honor. Each person speaks only when they are holding the Talking Stick. The Talking Stick is a powerful communication tool, which beautifully instills the skill of listening, being present, and tending to the moment.

In our world of overly scheduled calendars, mind-boggling technology, and expeditious modes of interacting, we seem to rely upon and expect accelerated communication in all respects. Yet, this paradigm does not translate so wonderfully into our more personal and intimate relationships. Efficiency, in this case, lacks depth and meaning.

Making a Talking Stick and then practicing using it can be a surprisingly powerful and meaningful way to enhance our skills in relating to one another. Using it slows everything down so that we can communicate with one another in a respectful and thoughtful way.

Lauren, Zach's preschool teacher, guided all of her four- and five-year-olds in making and then using a Talking Stick in the classroom. It was extraordinary to watch these children really listen to each other as they learned how to develop skills in cooperation and respecting one another. Each child then made a Talking Stick to bring home for the family.

Often it is Zach who will bring out the family Talking Stick when a disagreement is heading for a volcanic eruption. Using a talking stick doesn't necessarily mean you get what you want. But it does mean that you will be listened to, valued, and respected. Most of the time that is what is needed in the first place. I have found that using the Talking Stick opens me up more to the moment and being present with my child. When you listen carefully, you usually will discover that what you are warring over has little, if anything at all, to do with what may be going on with your child. The Talking Stick gives them a safe place to access their real feelings, thoughts, and ideas about their lives. Giving them respect teaches them how to be respectful, too.

The Talking Stick is an excellent tool to help parent and child work through difficult issues. As parents, we not only "teach" and model skills and qualities that we might deem "positive," but we also model for our children (consciously and unconsciously) ways in which to deal with conflict, stress, anger, fear, disappointment, or frustration. Our children are keen observers. So if you are feeling angry or frustrated about something that affects your child (directly or indirectly), communicate that appropriately in words. In doing so you honor your feelings while modeling for them how to honor their own. All in all, using the Talking Stick slows everything down and invites us to be totally in the moment, to be genuine in our communications and to listen, appreciate, and respect our loved ones.

MAKING THE TALKING STICK—First allow the youngest family member to choose a small branch or stick that may have been found in your yard or on a family walk or hike. (It can be anywhere from around twelve to twenty-four inches long and one-half to one inch or so in diameter). Bring the branch, embroidery thread, yarn or leather strap, beads, feathers, seashells, seeds, animal totem fetishes (any sacred objects you wish to decorate the branch with) to your *sacred space,* or to the place where you will be working together on creating the Talking Stick. Lay out all of the materials in the center of a table or on the floor. You can either talk about what you want to create together first, or close your eyes, listen to your favorite music together for a few minutes, and then allow the spirit of the Talking Stick or the music to move you.

Some people like to remove the bark by peeling or paring it off with a knife and then smoothing the wood with sandpaper. Others like to feel and see the natural texture of the branch. Select one end for the handle. Decorate the other end with your special materials. Since the Talking Stick belongs to the entire family, it is very important that everyone takes part in its creation.

Once made, bless it, smudge it, place it on the family altar or in a spot that is visible and accessible. Just being able to see the family Talking Stick is a reminder to practice good listening skills and work toward peaceful resolution. But don't forget to practice using it. That is where the best skills will be reenforced. If you practice enough, you will begin to recognize the cues (your child's and your own) that signal the rising of a potentially hurtful no-win battle. By appropriately intervening with the Talking Stick we guide ourselves back on track to where working toward a more productive resolution is possible. All in all, adapting the Talking Stick for our daily life cultivates tremendous skills in listening, being present, respecting and honoring each family member and the family as a whole.

Family Traditions Exercise

This exercise is meant to inspire, encourage, and to help you build upon whatever you might already be doing in your life, or to create something new and fresh. The idea is to integrate the meaningful or the spiritual into the flow of our ordinary life.

Have family members gather together in a special place (near the *family altar,* on the *sacred ground,* etc.) and write down all of the things that they find enjoyable (e.g., playing outside, taking walks, picnics, reading, baking). Once everyone has completed their list, select at least three things or have each family member pick one thing that everyone agrees upon. Either schedule it as a regular activity, or design it as a special ritual. The following are traditions suggested by friends.

Jeff and Gabe play basketball every Sunday morning with their friend Bob, who is in his early seventies. Gabe started going with his Dad to "pick-up" games when he was around two—that was five years ago.

Ken, Marilynn, and Zach take a family swim together every Sunday morning and then go out for bagels afterwards.

Create a reading circle, in which everyone in the family gets to read a poem or an excerpt from the book that they are currently reading.

Bake bread or make a pot of soup together once a week.

One family has agreed to do some kind of outdoor activity every Sunday afternoon (bike ride, take a walk, go to the zoo, have a picnic).

Steve and Zach have made pancakes together every Sunday morning since Zach was able to chew solid foods.

Write or videotape a family letter to a grandparent or relative who lives far away.

Plant and care for a family garden. Share your vegetables and flowers with someone special.

Play music together once a week.

Susan, David, and their three daughters make popcorn and watch a movie together every Friday night.

Create a quiet-time circle where each family member does something quietly—read, write, draw, meditate, stretch, or play with toys.

Light a candle and read from *A Grateful Heart* or *Enlightened Heart* (books with wonderful quotes) before having dinner.

When you have a family gathering create and tell a story together (I come from a family of quintessential storytellers who enjoy building a story—each child and adult can contribute a piece to the tale).

Keep a family journal that holds photographs, drawings, and notes to one another.

Order in pizza every Friday night and play a family game (Monopoly, charades, cards) or do a jigsaw puzzle.

Make a potluck dinner with other families once a month.

Pack a picnic lunch and take a walk to a park.

Many parks and zoos have programs where you can adopt a tree or an animal. Share in whatever responsibilities that may entail.

One Friday every month, one family cooks for an organization that delivers food to homebound individuals.

Every Saturday morning, Jeanne takes her nephew for a bus ride and a visit to the neighborhood fire station.

Kim and Lyn and their two children, Eli and Sydney, have created a notebook where once a week everyone shares something that they feel grateful for.

Take an evening walk with your children. Say good night to all of the creatures who live outdoors.

Look out the window every night and say good night to the moon.

One family loves to sing show tunes together.

Two sisters stay overnight at their grandmother's apartment and bake special breads.

Create a decorative piece for your kitchen table, front door, or family altar, from items found in nature.

Sponsor a child through a child services organization—write a family letter, create a special package to be mailed to the child every few weeks.

Every new or full moon, meditate together.

Sleep out under the stars in your backyard.

Create family meetings and projects (paint a room, plan an outing, talk about what is working, what is not, share appreciations).

Express gratitude regularly.

Sing, dance, and laugh together.

And don't forget to sing your child's song to him every chance you get.

Stories

The following stories express wonderful ways in which our children have been truly welcomed, honored, and loved by their family and community.

Traditional

- Many traditional cultures encourage young children to be in the company of their grandparents or other elders. They have much to teach each other, since they are both closer to the spirit world.

- For the Basque people in the Pyrenees, conception is a sacred act. From the moment of conception to puberty, the mother takes note of her dreams and impressions of the child, including specific events and stories. When the child reaches puberty, or a "marriageable age," the child's story is "given" (told) as a gift from mother to child.

- The Cherokee of the American Southwest believe that, "One always chooses their parents. . . .each of us has a sacred duty, a special gift that is necessary to the people who have chosen to be around us. We choose a family wherein our gifts may flourish, through which we can complete a cycle of learning. The most beautiful lesson that our elders taught us was not to rush, to know that everything flowers in its own time, and that each of us is a unique flower and cannot expect our blossom at the same time as another's. We were taught to respect variations."
- The Dagara of Africa believe that every child has a life's purpose. It is the duty of the entire village to help that child fulfill that purpose.

Personal
- One family honors their children's "firsts" (first day of school, losing the first tooth, first time flying on an airplane) with little celebrations. The celebration may include taking a photograph and then writing a letter to the child about the event (when they are older, children love to do this themselves). All of these letters, drawings, and photographs are kept together in an ongoing journal. The plan is to give these journals as gifts when the child turns eighteen.
- When his son was born, Kwabena, who is originally from central Ghana, called his mother to be given a name and a song for his child. Inspired by the day of the week he was born and the "cold and the rain" characteristic of of his birthplace in the Northwest, Kwabena's son is called Kwame (Saturday-born male) Bonsu (The whale in the rain). Kwabena sings his son's song to him when he is ill, hurts himself, on his birthday, and any time that he feels moved to celebrate and honor his child. Kwame Bonsu, now two, is often heard singing his own special song.

- The top of a weathered garden bench is what one family uses as their family altar. Beginning when their three children (around two years apart) were quite little, each family member brought something that was important to them (flowers, a book, a photograph, a toy truck, a tiny squishy bear) to put on the altar. The "sacred objects" change from time to time.

- Elijah, age five, says that sitting on her grandma Linda's lap is her "most favorite place to sit in all of the world, because it is so safe there."

- An old pine blanket chest has evolved into our family altar. Having held my favorite books, it has now become a "lap" for candles, seashells, stones, a tree branch, Zach's beaded baby moccasins, and my personal favorite—a musical Kermit the Frog. When I place my faded Southwestern Indian blanket on the floor, in front of the chest, I create what I call my *sacred ground*. It is where I meditate, perform rituals, and sometimes hang out with Zach. Occasionally while sitting on our *sacred ground*, Zach will tell or write a story.

RITUALS, CEREMONIES, AND CELEBRATIONS

Part of creating a life with more meaning is to practice acknowledging the preciousness of the moment. Designing and participating in rituals, ceremonies, and celebrations is one of the ways in which we can begin to notice and appreciate the extraordinary in the ordinary.

Beginning Anew

This ritual is inspired by a ceremony practiced weekly at Plum Village, a meditation community in southwestern France where Thich Nhat Hanh lives. Its purpose is to express and clear feelings that might otherwise build up over time. The ceremony is structured in three parts: flower-watering (genuinely acknowledging the wonderful qualities of others), expressing regrets, and sharing hurts and difficulties. This ritual can be tremendously beneficial to our own families if practiced regularly, ideally once a week.

Come together once a week in your *sacred place,* or anywhere you feel comfortable. Sit in a circle and place a vase of fresh flowers in its center. Light a candle. When someone wishes to speak, she stands, walks slowly to the flowers, takes the vase in her hands, and returns to her seat. She is allowed as much time as she needs to acknowledge and express her appreciation for the whole family or someone in particular. Everyone else practices deep *listening.* When she is finished expressing her feelings, she stands up and slowly returns the vase to the center of the circle.

In the second part of the ceremony, anyone can express regrets for anything that they may have done or said to hurt others during the past week. This offers an opportunity to recall a regret or heal a wound that may have been inflicted during the week.

In the third part of the ceremony, express ways in which you feel others may have hurt you. This ceremony is not about judging, arguing, or blaming. Speak truthfully, but not destructively.

Beginning Anew offers a sacred venue for expressing our feelings, while at the same time cultivates a keener awareness and understanding about our dynamics of relating (to ourselves and to our loved ones). All in all, through compassionate listening, honoring, and respecting one another, we heal and strengthen the family's soul.

Close the ceremony with a song and a family hug.

Welcoming the Family Soul

Just as in *Welcoming the Soul of a Child Ritual,* this ceremony and celebration is meant to honor not only the birth, but the ongoing life of the family soul. The main purpose of the ritual is to create a regular practice of honoring and nourishing the family. If you wish you can include *Welcoming the Soul of the Family Meditation* as part of the ceremony.

What you will need: a potted plant or tree, a small pitcher of water, and any ceremonial items that you would like to use (e.g., vase of flowers, candle, cushions, blanket, meditation bell, or chimes).

Prepare your ceremonial space (lay out a blanket and cushions, purify the space, create an altar). Ringing a meditation bell, running your fingers through wind chimes, or playing a musical instrument (a drum or triangle, for example) can be a lovely signal to your children that the ritual is beginning. Once seated in a circle, take a moment for silence (to still our minds and bodies, so that we can be fully present). Then have each member express anything that they feel they need to share. Think, in particular, about where the family can use more nourishment (more quiet time together, more time to laugh and be silly, cleaning a room or a closet, listening to each other better, weeding the garden). Also think about something that you appreciate about the family or a family member (how everyone helped in preparing a meal, a walk that you just took together, someone being kind or forgiving). After the sharing, move closer around the potted plant or tree. Each person takes a turn watering the tree (from the pitcher of water being passed around) while saying a prayer silently or out loud. Or as a family you might write something together that expresses the symbolism of tenderly caring for this tree ("May the roots of this tree receive the proper nutrients to allow for sturdy and secure growth. May its branches continue to stretch toward the heavens, while remaining deeply connected to Mother Earth, to all of her wisdom . . ."). Bring the ceremony to a close with a story, a song, or a quote or blessing from a favorite book. Conclude with a family hug.

Note: You can also adapt this ritual by incorporating a favorite tree found in your yard, in a park, or in the woods. (Read *Nature as a Teacher* in this chapter about selecting a *Guardian Tree*).

THE SOUL SONG: THE UNCUT VERSION

Two weeks before Zach's due date, I had my last session with Carol, a licensed chiropractor and a wonderful energy healer. Since I'd begun working with her in my fifth month, Carol would sometimes share what she was intuitively feeling from the baby. On this particular day, I asked Carol if she was sensing anything from Zach. She softly said, "I feel he is wanting you to know that if the birth doesn't go as you might hope, it has no connection with what you have or haven't done. It will be more about what he is needing for his own coming and spiritual growth."

I felt a chill to my bones. Although I had invited the information, it didn't buffer the fear that shot to the surface. What exactly did this mean? Hadn't I done all of the things that I was "supposed" to do—select an ob-gyn I trusted, eat properly, draw up a Birth Plan, exercise daily, dutifully ingest my prenatal vitamins, practice meditation and visualizations for labor and birth, listen to music, sing lullabies, talk and write to my baby, etc., etc.? I struggled to reconcile honoring Zach's wish or destiny with what I felt was my responsibility to make the birth experience as natural and as positive as possible for both of us.

The next day, Zach, who had been in the "perfect position," flipped over on his back. After getting through early morning sickness, I had been blessed with a blissful pregnancy. I absolutely loved being pregnant. I loved knowing that Zach and I were dancing this exquisite dance together and was excited about the new waltz or tango that we were practicing for the

Big Day. But once he swan dived into the "head and body pressing up against my spine" position, everything seemed to shift. I was becoming mentally, physically, and emotionally uncomfortable, and I wondered if he was, too.

I continued to meditate, take walks, and dialogue with my unborn son (via nondominant handwriting and meditation). I felt assured that the birth experience would be what was needed for both Zach and me. I began to let go of my vision of what I thought the birth experience was "supposed" to look like and tried to turn it over to the larger forces co-producing this event.

Zach was born two days before his due date by c-section after more than eighteen hours of excruciating back labor. The support of my husband, family, and friends helped me recover from the surgery very quickly. However, the emotional scarring took much longer to heal. Despite my heartfelt attempt to honor the "message" and the unexpected, a part of me felt as though I had let everyone down, most of all my newborn. Once settled in at home with Zachary, I gradually began to do the healing work that seemed to be required of me at this particular time in my life.

Whether what Carol had accessed that day was Zach's wisdom, my own, or hers—or whether we all had somehow broadcast a simultaneous news bulletin—does not seem as important as how both Zach and I were and are healing. Our experience has definitely asked me to heal deeper wounds, the depths of which I was not even aware before his birth.

At the time, I wondered if the message from Zach was really telling me that this particular birth experience was necessary for his soul's growth and evolution. Or were all of the fine details of the birth influenced by my beliefs, attitudes, and unresolved issues? By letting me know ahead of time, maybe Zach was trying to appease my need to do everything right and take full responsibility if it wasn't, no matter the circumstances. Or maybe it was just a random occurrence, a folding and overlapping of the unknown. Perhaps it was a combination of all of the above. I'll never know.

What I do know is that it is vitally important to me to continue my personal healing work. Only from this place will I be able to truly *listen* for Zachary's soul song. For you see, as I grow as a mother, I also am beginning to understand that genuinely *listening* means honoring and respecting the whole song—the whole child—most especially when the melody and tone might sound discordant and disturbing to my ears.

A friend directed me to the following story when I found myself grappling with this idea of welcoming and honoring our child's soul song in its entirety—not just the version that we might give a fabulous review.

One summer, while trekking through Nepal on the north-eastern slopes of Annapurna, poet David Whyte came upon an ancient monastery. With Buddhism declining in this particular region, the monastery had been neglected and was now decaying. Everything inside, however, had remained exactly as it always had been. Entering into the monastery from the brilliant, clear light of the snowy slopes, Whyte found himself in total darkness. As his eyes slowly adjusted, the very first thing that he saw was a statue of the fierce Guardian Deity—a terrifying-looking statue with skulls around its neck and blood dripping from its fangs, crushing someone with his clawed feet and holding a spear pointed directly at all those who entered.

Traditionally the Guardian Deity's message is interpreted as "You need to leave all of your fears behind!" Whyte, however, was struck by another thought: "Be sure that you bring your fears with you. All of you has to enter, especially your fears, your flaws, the parts that you are scared of and have disowned." He firmly believes that the Buddha invites us to enter leaving no part of ourselves behind. "After all," he observed at the monastery, "as you look beyond the spear, you can clearly see into the shrine room where the Buddha beckons you."

Just as the Beloved Buddha beckons all aspects of the individual to enter into the sacred shrine, we, when inviting our children to join us, need to welcome, greet, honor, and love all of who they are, to embrace their whole beingness. For I believe that intrinsic to each and every child's song is a myriad of sounds and vibrations; ranging from light, playful, and sweet to dark, thunderous, ominous, and raging. I am certain, however, that we will be unable to embrace them in this way, unless we are willing to appreciate and understand our own discordant notes.

Being devoted to our healing journey and allowing our soul to cry, grieve, howl, laugh, sing, and dance can help to strengthen and expand our capacity to be more present to all of our life. When we are able to genuinely and authentically meet ourselves, we create the sacred ground where we can come and meet our child—eye to eye, heart to heart, and soul to soul. Not a simple day's work. But what have we taken life for, if not to grow, heal, unfold, and love ourselves and our children into being?

> *We are because we are seen;*
> *We are because we are loved,*
> *The world is because it is beheld*
> *and loved into being.*
> —ANITA BARROWS

SINGING AND DANCING IN THE GARDEN

On a writing retreat one fall, I stayed on one of those ravishing islands found in the Pacific Northwest. It was there that I came across a hand-carved stone polar bear that literally took my breath away. I was enchanted by how movement, beauty, and grace were beautifully expressed through the smooth polished granite. Just looking at it made me smile.

I was told that the carving had been crafted by a very talented Inuit Indian living in the Northwest Territory, and that the piece had a name, Dancing Bear. It turns out that Dancing Bear is a theme used by many Inuit carvers who live in the region.

You see, the inspiration comes from real life. Besides observing the bears giving each other affectionate hugs and bites, rolling around on the ice and snow, the Inuit people have seen the bears climb up on steep slippery snowbanks and then slide down them, over and over again—apparently all in the spirit of fun! And this is the best part: It has been reported that some lucky people have seen those magnificent fluffs of fur and strength balance all several thousand pounds of themselves on one foot—and dance!

I thought, perhaps we all need a dancing bear carving around to remind us to play. But then, a moment later, I realized we do have a reminder. . . .every day. Our children are our Dancing Bears. We just need to slow down our pace, take one of their paws, and dance!

Singing and dancing in the garden is a dynamic celebration of our soul's work. In doing our inner healing, we naturally begin to integrate the fragmented and disowned parts of ourselves. When we "invite these aspects of ourself in for tea," or take them in our arms and waltz, we begin to embrace our whole being, thus allowing us to fully embrace our child. In healing our soul wounds, we create a canvas for expressing our soul's gifts, right along with our child's.

Our children's open heart, genuine dynamic spirit, and sheer ravishing beauty stirs us out of our deep trancelike sleep, inviting us to take off our shoes and dance—to get in touch with our own "wild child," to *listen* for our soul's song.

However, even when the garden is flourishing in its fullest

bloom, we need to remain constant in practicing our cultivated skills, for at any time we can easily be lulled back into that dark sleep. Even the most sturdy and hearty plants will die from neglect or be smothered by an overly protective and unaware hand.

> *The breeze of dawn has secrets to tell you.*
> *Don't go back to sleep.*
> *You must ask for what you really want.*
> *Don't go back to sleep.*
> *People are going back and forth*
> *Across the doors where*
> *The two worlds touch.*
> *The door is round and open*
> *Do not go back to sleep.*
>
> —RUMI

The great Persian poet Rumi urges us not to slip back into the trancelike sleep. If we do, we miss the "secrets" that "the breeze of dawn" wishes to tell us, or singing and dancing with our child, sharing in their sense of wonder and fully feeling their soul's song open and touch the world. We miss an eternity of simple moments, pure and light—slipping away unnoticed. When we are fully awake we can, paradoxically, close our eyes, move into the stillness and hear ... a chorus of voices singing, voices that connect us to the music of the spheres, to the majesty and mystery of life, to the depths of ourselves and to one another. And we will hear the souls of our children singing, *"LISTEN ..."*

Coda

It's autumn, my favorite season. We are letting go of the lush greens and welcoming the translucent golds and fiery reds. These vibrant tones of change move all around us.

We, too, are moving. My husband, son, and I are moving to a new home. And as I sort through our belongings, I reflect on how blessed we have been. Many changes have been seeded here, some that have come to fruition and some that have not. Yet certainly, the most meaningful change has been the conception and arrival of our son, Zach.

Zach was conceived one bright crisp autumn morning—very much like this one. My husband, Steve, and I had lighted a rose-scented candle, whispered a prayer, and while slipping under our flannel sheets, invited the child into our life—into our world.

This wasn't the first time that we had called out to the spirit of a child. In fact, for a number of years prior to living in our nineteenth-century farmhouse, we had tried to become pregnant. An ovulation kit packed with our vacation clothes traveled with us from the Caribbean to the Rockies. To our surprise, pregnancy didn't come easily, and when it did, it was terminated spontaneously (three times).

The miscarriages brought both physical and emotional pain and became the catalyst for an outward and inward exploration. Neither the experts nor our loved ones ever discouraged us from trying again, but after the last miscarriage, my husband and I decided to take a breather. We would rest and then talk about how we might proceed.

Interestingly, it was during that space of breathing that Zach came to us—soaring into our world with his very own life force—dramatic and spirited.

For some reason, we had been inspired to make love that morning in one of our guest bedrooms, the bedroom that became Zach's—or perhaps, more truthfully said, the bedroom that was his all along, but merely waiting for him—much like his parents.

Imbued as it was with the essences of new life blended with the old, you might understand why this particular home holds the treasures that it does for us. Many magical moments occurred here in the beginnings of Zach's life. It seemed natural and important to leave a gift thanking the house for its blessings. So one day we planted a little white pine tree. The pine joined the towering locusts and maples that had watched over this land and home for several hundred years. Together they stood on the gentle hillside while we held hands around the tree's delicate branches, saying our prayer of thanks to our home.

A few days later, taking a break from the arduous task of packing, Zach and I shared a toasted cinnamon bagel at our favorite cafe. I asked Zach what he thought about our ensuing move. He quietly replied, "I don't like it much." "Do you think you'll miss our house, Zachy?" I inquired. "Yeah," he softly said, gazing down at his uneaten bagel. Feeling the need to comfort him, yet honor his feelings, I shared that I, too, would miss our wonderful old house, even though I was looking forward to the move. He then asked if the same moon that we searched for in the night sky as part of our night-time ritual could be found outside his bedroom window at the new house. "Oh, yes," I responded, moved by the question. "The same moon will be at both houses?" Now he sounded a tiny bit reassured. I nodded a big "um hm." "Oh," he sighed. "So the moon will watch over the farmhouse and the little tree, even after we move? That's nice."

I offer this book to you and to your children as a way to create and discover for yourself how to honor your life and the lives of your children. And as the moon watches over the little trees, may we be faithful in our commitment to watch over our children and to see the sacredness in our role as parents. Let this be a caring reminder to listen ever so keenly to your child's individual song—to sing it to them and with them, tenderly and lovingly, throughout the days and nights of their lives. Perhaps we then might all come together to hear a symphony of songs under the same moon amongst the sacred trees.

Index of Exercises and Rituals

This Index is created for easy access to the exercises, rituals, ceremonies, and celebrations offered throughout the book. They are listed according to subject. Remember to think of what is offered as a reservoir of possibilities. Choose which ones are relevant to you, your baby, family and community of friends.

Communing With Your Baby and Child

Inner Journey Healing

Couples/Relationship Healing

Family/Community

Visualizations/Creative Imagery

Meditations/Being Present

Recommended Reading

The following books and resources are offered for additional information, support, and encouragement during all of the various stages of *birthing* a child and a family.

Bonding and Communicating with Your Unborn Child

Bonding before Birth: A Guide to Becoming a Family, Leni Schwartz (Salem, MA: Sigo Press, 1991).

The Child of Your Dreams: Approaching Conception and Pregnancy with Inner Peace and Reverence for Life to Enhance the Development of Your Future Child, Laura Archera Huxley and Piero Ferrucci (Rochester, VT: Destiny Books, 1992).

Communing with the Spirit of Your Unborn Child, Dawson Church (Boulder Creek, CA: Aslan Publishing, 1988).

Continuum Concept, Jean Liedloff (Reading, MA: Addison-Wesley, 1986).

Cradle from Heaven: Psychological and Spiritual Dimensions of Conception, Pregnancy and Birth, Murshida Vera Justin Corda (Lebanon Springs, NY: Omega Press, 1987).

Diary of an Unborn Child: An Unborn Baby Speaks to its Mother, Manuel David Coudris (Bath, ENG: Gateway Books, 1992).

Love Start: Learn to Communicate with Your Unborn Baby and Take Charge of Your Child's Birth, Eve Marnie (Carson, CA: Hay House, 1989).

The Mind of Your Newborn Baby, David Chamberlain (Berkeley: North Alantic Books, 1998).

Nurturing the Unborn Child: A Nine-Month Program for Soothing, Stimulating, and Communicating with Your Baby, Thomas Verny, M.D., and Pamela Weintraub (New York: Bantam Doubleday Dell, 1991).

Primal Connections: How our Experiences from Conception to Birth Influence our Emotions, Behavior, and Health, Elizabeth Noble (New York: Simon & Schuster, 1993).

The Secret Life of The Unborn Child, Thomas Verny, M.D., and John Kelley (New York: Dell, 1982).

Soul Trek: Meeting our Children on the Way to Birth, Elisabeth Hallett (Manilton, MT: Light Hearts Publishing, 1995).

The Tibetan Art of Parenting: From before Conception through Early Childhood, Anne Hubbell Maiden and Edie Farwell (Somerville, MA: Wisdom, 1997).

Pregnancy and Birthing

Adoption: A Handful of Hope, Suzanne Arms (Berkeley, CA: Celestial Arts, 1990).

A Birth Partner's Handbook: How to Help a Woman through Childbirth, Carl Jones with Jan Jones (New York: Simon & Schuster, 1989).

Birthing Normally: A Personal Growth Approach to Childbirth, 2nd ed., Gayle Peterson (Berkeley, CA: Shadow & Light Publications, 1984).

A Child Is Born, Linnart Neilsson (New York: Delacorte, 1990).

A Good Birth, a Safe Birth, Diana Korte and Roberta Scaer (New York: Bantam Books, 1984).

After the Baby's Birth . . . A Woman's Way to Wellness: A Complete Guide for Postpartum Women, Robin Lim (Berkeley, CA: Celestial Arts, 1991).

After the Baby Is Born: A Complete Postpartum Guide for New Parents, Carl Jones (New York: Henry Holt & Co., 1986).

Alternative Birth: The Complete Guide, Carl Jones (Los Angeles, CA: Jeremy PI Tarcher, Inc., 1991).

Birth Reborn, Michel Odent (Illinois: Livingstone, 1994).

Birth Without Violence, Frederick Leboyer (Rochester, VT: Healing Arts, 1975/1996).

Childbirth with Insight, Elizabeth Noble (Boston: Houghton-Mifflin, 1983).

Childbirth Without Fear, rev. ed., Grantly Dick-Read (New York: Harper, 1944/1994).

Complete Book of Pregnancy and Childbirth, Sheila Kitzinger (New York: Knopf, rev. 1989).

Creating a Joyful Birth Experience, Lucia Capacchione and Sandra Bardsley (New York: Simon & Schuster, 1994).

The Creative Journal for Parents, Lucia Capacchione (Boston: Shambhala, book in progress).

An Easier Childbirth: A Mother's Workbook for Health and Emotional Well-Being during Pregnancy and Delivery, Gayle Peterson (Berkeley: Shadow & Light, 1993).

Gentle Birth Choices, Barbara Harper (Rochester, VT: Healing Arts Press, 1994).

Having Twins: A Parent's Guide to Pregnancy, Birth and Early Childhood, 2nd ed., Elizabeth Noble (Boston: Houghton Mifflin, 1990).

Immaculate Deception II: Myth, Magic & Birth, Suzanne Arms (Berkeley, CA: Celestial Arts, 1996).

Infant Massage: A Handbook for Loving Parents, Vimala Schneider McClure (New York: Bantam, 1989).

The Language Of Fertility: A Revolutionary Mind-Body Program For Conscious Conception, Niravi B. Payne, M.S., and Brenda Lane Richardson (New York: Harmony Books, 1997).

The Lesbian and Gay Parenting Handbook, April Martin (New York: Harper Collins, 1993).

Loving Hands: The Traditional Indian Art of Baby Massaging, Frederick LeBoyer (New York: Knopf, 1976).

Mind Over Labor: How to Reduce the Fear and Pain of Childbirth through Mental Imagery, Carl Jones (New York: Viking/Penguin, 1987).

Motherprayer: The Pregnant Woman's Spiritual Companion, Tikva Frymer-Kensky (New York: Riverhead Books, 1995).

Mothering The Mother: How a Doula Can Help You Have a Shorter, Easier, and Healthier Birth, John Kennell, Marshall H. Klaus, and Phyllis Klaus (Reading, MA: Addison-Wesley/Lawrence, 1993).

Mothering the New Mother, Sally Placksin (New York: Newmarket Press, 1994).

The Nature Of Birth And Breastfeeding, Michel Odent (Westport, CT: Bergin & Garvey, 1992).

The Nurturing Father, Kyle D. Pruett, M.D. (New York: Warner, 1987).

Positive Pregnancy Fitness, Sylvia Klein Olkin (New York: Avery Publishers, 1987).

Pregnancy as Healing: Holistic Philosophy for Prenatal Care, Gayle Peterson and Lewis Mehl (Berkeley, CA: Mindbody Press, 1984).

Pregnancy, Childbirth and the Newborn, Penny Simkin, Janet Whalley, and Ann Keppler (Deerhaven, MN: Meadowbrook Press, 1991).

Pregnant Fathers: Entering Parenthood Together, Jack Heinowitz (San Diego, CA: Parents As Partner Press, 1994).

Pregnant Feelings: Developing Trust In Birth, Rahima Baldwin and Terra Palmarinir Richardson (Berkeley: Celestial Arts, 1986).

The Pregnant Woman's Comfort Book: A Self-Nurturing Guide to Your Emotional Well-Being during Pregnancy and Early Motherhood, Jennifer Louden (New York: Harper-Collins, 1995).

The Primal Wound: Understanding the Adopted Child, Nancy Newton Verrier (Baltimore, MD: Gateway Press, 1997).

Special Delivery: The Complete Guide to Informed Birth, Rahima Baldwin (Berkeley, CA: Celestial Arts, 1990).

The Tao Of Motherhood, Vimala McClure (Willow Springs, MO: Nucleus, 1991).

Visualizations for an Easier Childbirth, Carl Jones (New York: Simon & Schuster, 1988).

The Well Baby Book, Mike Samuels and Nancy Samuels (New York: Simon & Schuster, 1991).

The Well Pregnancy Book, Mike Samuels and Nancy Samuels (New York: Simon & Schuster, 1996).

When Men Are Pregnant, Jerold Lee Shapiro, Ph.D. (New York: Delta, 1987).

The Year after Childbirth, Sheila Kitzinger (New York: Scribners, 1994).

Your Amazing Newborn, Marshall H. Klaus, Phyllis H. Klaus (Reading, MA: Perseus Books, 1998).

Your Baby, Your Way: Making Pregnancy Decisions and Birth Plans, Sheila Kitzinger (New York: Pantheon, 1987).

Water Birth: Dispelling the Myth—Embracing the Magic, Barbara Harper (Rochester, VT: Healing Arts Press, book in progress).

We Are All Water Babies, Jessica Johnson and Michel Odent (Berkeley, CA: Celestial Arts, 1995).

A Wise Birth: Bringing Together The Best Of Natural Childbirth With Modern Medicine, Penny Armstrong and Sheryl Feldman (New York: William Morrow, 1990).

Women's Bodies, Women's Wisdom: Creating Physical and Emotional Health and Healing, Christiane Northrup (New York: Bantam, 1994).

Parenting

Celebrating The Great Mother: A Handbook of Earth-Honoring Activities for Parents and Children, Cait Johnson and Maura D. Shaw (Rochester, VT: Destiny Books, 1995).

The Creative Journal for Parents, Lucia Capacchione (Boston: Shambhala, book in progress).

Everyday Blessings: The Inner Work of Mindful Parenting, Myla and Jon Kabat-Zinn (New York: Hyperion, 1997).

The Geography of Childhood: Why Children Need Wild Places, Gary Paul Nabhan and Stephen Trimble (Boston: Beacon Press, 1994).

The Joyful Child: A Sourcebook of Activities and Ideas for Releasing Children's Natural Joy, Peggy Jenkins, Ph.D. (Santa Rosa, CA: Aslan Publishing, 1996).

The Lesbian and Gay Parenting Handbook, April Martin (New York: HarperCollins, 1993).

Models of Love: The Parent-Child Journey, Barry Vissell, M.D., and Joyce Vissell (Aptos, CA: Ramira Publishing, 1986).

Raising an Emotionally Intelligent Child: The Heart of Parenting, John Gottman (New York, NY: Simon & Schuster, 1997).

Sharing Nature with Children, Joseph Cornell (Nevada City, CA: Dawn Publications, 1998).

Spiritual Parenting: A Sourcebook for Parents and Teachers, Steven M. Rosman, Ph.D., MSC. (Wheaton, IL: The Theosophical Publishing House, 1994).

The Tibetan Art Of Parenting: From before Conception through Early Childhood, Anne Hubbell Maiden and Edie Farwell (Somerville, MA: Wisdom Publications, 1997).

Whole Child/Whole Parent, Polly Berrien Berends (New York: HarperCollins, 1987).

Wonderful Ways to Love a Child, Judy Ford (Berkeley, CA: Conari Press, 1997).

Inner Healing

Birthing Normally: A Personal Growth Approach to Childbirth, 2nd ed., Gayle Peterson (Berkeley, CA: Shadow & Light Publications, 1984).

The Creative Journal, Lucia Capacchione (North Hollywood: New Castle Publishing Co., Inc., 1989).

Dancing Up the Moon: A Woman's Guide to Creating Traditions that Bring Sacredness to Daily Life, Robin Heerens Lysne (Berkeley, CA: Conari Press, 1995).

Ended Beginings: Healing Childbearing Losses, Claudia Panuthos and Catherine Romeo (South Hadley, MA: Bergin and Garvey, 1984).

Essence: The Diamond Approach to Inner Realization, A.H. Almaas (York Beach, Maine: Samuel Weiser, Inc., 1986).

Good Grief Rituals, Elaine Childs-Gowell, Ph.D. (Barrytown, NY: Station Hill Press, 1992).

Guided Meditations, Explorations and Healings, Stephen Levine (New York: Anchor Books, 1991).

Healing into Life and Death, Stephen Levine (New York: Doubleday, 1979, 1989). (Includes powerful healing meditation—"Opening the Heart of the Womb", which can be ordered on audio cassette from: Warm Rocks Tapes, P.O. Box 108, Chamisal, New Mexico 87521. Or call 1-800-731-HEAL.)

The Language Of Fertility: A Revolutionary Mind-Body Program for Conscious Conception, Niravi B. Payne, M.S., and Brenda Lane Richardson (New York: Harmony Books, 1997).

Minding the Body, Mending the Mind, Joan Borysenko (New York: Bantam Books, 1987).

The Picture of Health: Healing Your Life with Art, Lucia Capacchione (Carson, CA: Hay House, 1992).

The Soul Wound, Thomas Yeomans (The Concord Institute, Box 82, Concord, MA: (978) 371-3206).

The Well Being Journal, Lucia Capacchione (North Hollywood, CA: Newcastle, 1989).

What We May Be: Techniques for Psychological and Spiritual Growth through Psychosynthesis, Piero Ferrucci (New York: G.P. Putnam's Sons, 1982).

The Woman's Comfort Book: A Self-Nurturing Guide for Restoring Balance in Your Life, Jennifer Louden (New York: HarperCollins, 1992).

Womanspirit: A Guide to Women's Wisdom, Hallie Austen Iglehart (San Francisco: Harper & Row, 1993).

Transformation through Birth: A Woman's Guide, Claudia Panuthos (Westport, CT: Greenwood Publishing Group, 1984).

Couples/Relationships

Embracing the Beloved: Relationship as a Path of Awakening, Stephen and Ondrea Levine (New York: Bantam, 1995).

The Couple's Comfort Book: A Creative Guide for Renewing Passion, Pleasure & Commitment, Jennifer Louden (New York: HarperCollins, 1994).

Journey of the Heart: Intimate Relationship and the Path of Love, John Welwood, Ph.D. (New York: HarperCollins, 1990).

Love and Awakening: Discovering the Sacred Path of Intimate Relationship, John Welwood (New York: HarperCollins, 1996).

The Shared Heart: Relationship, Inititations and Celebration, Barry Vissell, M.D., and Joyce Vissell (Oakland, CA: Ramira Publishing, 1984).

The Spirit Of Intimacy: Ancient Teaching in the Ways of Relationships, Sobonfu E. Somé (Berkeley, CA: Berkeley Hills Books, 1997).

The Unimaginable Life: Lessons Learned on the Path of Love, Kenny and Julia Loggins (New York, NY 1997).

Being Present/Mindfulness

A Gradual Awakening, Stephen Levine (New York: Anchor Books, Doubleday, 1979, 1989).

A Path with Heart: A Guide through the Perils and Promises of Spiritual Life, Jack Kornfield (New York: Bantam Books, 1993).

Buddha's Little Instruction Book, Jack Kornfield (New York: Bantam Books, 1994).

LovingKindness, Sharon Salzberg (Boston: Shambhala, 1995).

Peace Is Every Step: The Path of Mindfulness in Everyday Life, Thich Nhat Hanh (New York: Bantam Books, 1991).

Teachings on Love, Thich Nhat Hanh (Berkeley, CA: Parallax Press, 1997).

Wherever You Go, There You Are, Jon Kabat-Zinn (New York: St. Martin's Press, 1994).

Videotapes

Body-Centered Hypnosis for Childbirth, Gayle Peterson. Shadow & Light Productions, 1749 Vine Street, Berkeley, CA 94703.

Comfort Measures for Childbirth, Penny Simkin. 1100 23rd Avenue East, Seattle, WA 98112. (206) 324-5440.

Gentle Birth Choices, Barbara Harper. Global Maternal/Child Health Association, Inc. P.O. Box 1400, Wilsonville, OR 97070. (503) 682-3600.

Resources

ASSOCIATION FOR PRENATAL AND PERINATAL
PSYCHOLOGY (APPPAH)
340 Colony Road
Box 994
Geyserville, CA 95441
(707) 857-4041
Email: apppah@aol.com
Website: http://www.birthpsychology.com
Organization founded by Thomas Verny, M.D., dedicated to in-
depth exploration of the psychological, emotional, and social
development of babies and parents from preparation for preg-
nancy through the postpartum period.

BIRTH AND LIFE BOOKSTORE
141 Commercial Street NE
Salem, OR 97301
(800) 736-0631
(503) 371-4445
Email onecascade@worldnet.att.net
Website: Icascade.com
This complete mail-order business offers extensive catalogues on
book, pamphlets, videos, and personal and professional supplies
related to conception, pregnancy, birth, babies, midwifery, parenting, and nutrition.

DOULAS OF NORTH AMERICA (DONA)
1100 23rd Avenue East
Seattle, WA 98112
(206) 324-5440

INTERNATIONAL CESAREAN AWARENESS
NETWORK (ICAN)
P.O. Box 276
Clarks Summit, PA 18411
(717) 585-4226
Provides information on preventing unnecessary cesareans, planning for VBACs (vaginal birth after caesarian), and helping women to recover from traumatic births.

LA LECHE LEAGUE INTERNATIONAL
1400 North Meacham Road
Schaumburg, IL 60173-4840
(800) LA LECHE (For questions related to breastfeeding)
(847) 519-7730 (Catalogue of books and resources;
directory of articles and other materials available from
the La Leche League Reference Library and Database)
Email: Illhq@ill.org
Website: http://www.laleague.org/

GLOBAL MATERNAL/CHILD HEALTH
ASSOCIATION, INC.
P.O. Box 1400
Wilsonville, Oregon 97070
(503) 682-3600
Email: waterbirth@aol.com
Website: www.geocities.com/hotsprings/2840
Founded by Barbara Harper *(Gentle Birth Choices*/book and video), which is dedicated to education and research about natural childbirth, including the use of water to ease labor and birth. Has most recent list of hospitals throughout the U.S.A. that authorize water births. Also rents and sells birthing tubs.

MIDWIVES ALLIANCE OF NORTH AMERICA (MANA)
P.O. Box 1121
Bristol, VA 24203
(615) 764-5561

PEPS (Program For Early Parent Support)
4649 Sunnyside Avenue North, #346
Seattle, WA 98103-6900
(206) 547-8570
Email: pepsgroup@aol.com
PEPS is a nonprofit service organization based in Seattle, WA, which supports parents of infants and young children. A replication package is available for starting a PEPS program in your community.

WHOLE PERSON FERTILITY PROGRAM
Niravi B. Payne, M.S.
100 Remsen Street
Brooklyn, NY 11201
(718) 625-4802
(800) 666-HEALTH
Email: niravi@aol.com

WILDERNESS AWARENESS SCHOOL
26331 N.E. Valley Street
#5-147
Duvall, WA 98019
(425-788-1301)
Email: wasnet@natureoutlet.com
Website: www.NatureOutlet.com
Wilderness Awareness School, founded by Jon Young, is a school devoted to teaching individuals of all ages how to reconnect with the wisdom found in nature.

Permissions

Dear Reader,

It is through the telling of our stories that we are reminded just how connected we truly are. If you would like to share your story or any comments regarding this book, I invite you to contact me.

With gratitude,

Jill

soulsong@wolfenet.com
P.O. Box 31962, Seattle, WA 98103